PALEO D

C000257186

Easy, Healthy and Delicious Paleolithic Recipes for a Nourishing Meal

(Everything You Need to Know About Paleo Diet)

Steven Rodriguez

Published by Alex Howard

Steven Rodriguez

Paleo Diet: Easy, Healthy and Delicious Paleolithic Recipes for a Nourishing Meal (Everything You Need to Know About Paleo Diet)

ISBN 978-1-77485-027-5

Legal & Disclaimer

The information contained in this book is not designed to replace or take the place of any form of medicine or professional medical advice. The information in this book has been provided for educational and entertainment purposes only.

The information contained in this book has been compiled from sources deemed reliable, and it is accurate to the best of the Author's knowledge; however, the Author cannot guarantee its accuracy and validity and cannot be held liable for any errors or omissions. Changes are periodically made to this book. You must consult your doctor or get professional medical advice before using any of the suggested remedies, techniques, or information in this book.

Upon using the information contained in this book, you agree to hold harmless the Author from and against any damages, costs, and expenses, including any legal fees potentially resulting from the application of any of the information provided by this guide. This disclaimer applies to any damages or injury caused by the use and application, whether directly or indirectly, of any advice or information presented, whether for breach of contract, tort, negligence, personal injury, criminal intent, or under any other cause of action.

You agree to accept all risks of using the information presented inside this book. You need to consult a professional medical practitioner in order to ensure you are both able and healthy enough to participate in this program.

Table of Contents

Part 1

Introduction

This book has tasty Paleo recipes to help you lose weight.

In the recent past, there has been a lot of talk about the paleo diet and the amazing benefits you can enjoy by simply going Paleo. One of the most talked about benefits of going on a paleo diet is weight loss. I assure you that the Paleo diet is nothing like a fad diet but is instead a way of living. Therefore, if you are only looking to lose a few pounds and get back to your bad eating habits, then the paleo diet is not for you.

If you want to learn more about the paleo diet, what it is, how to lose weight while on the diet and some amazing recipes, then this book has just that and much more. You will learn what to eat and what not to eat on a paleo diet and why. You will also have access to over 20 tasty paleo recipes that are easy to make. Trust me, with this book, losing weight has never been easier.

Thanks again for downloading this book, I hope you enjoy it!

The Paleo Diet Basics

Before we can move on and have a look at some tasty paleo recipes, it is crucial to understand what the paleo diet is, what to eat while on a paleo diet, and how it can help you lose weight.

For starters, the paleo diet entails eating what the paleolithic man ate; this is before invent of agriculture. The then man ate wild fruits, herbs, game meat and wild caught fish. This is very different from what the current man eats. Nowadays, we cannot go a day without eating wheat, taking unhealthy fats and drinking beverages high in sugar. It is no wonder that the modern man is plagued with many diseases such as high blood pressure, diabetes, heart disease, and obesity. Since your goal is to lose weight, how can going on a paleo diet make you lose weight?

While on a paleo diet, you focus on eating real food like fruits, green leafy vegetables, game meat and wild caught fish, which is a healthier diet as compared to eating French fries, potato chips, cakes, cookies, candies, and soda. Since you will not be eating these foods, which are quite high in empty calories, this greatly reduces the amount of calories you eat; hence, automatic weight loss. With that in mind, let us look at what to eat and avoid while on a paleo diet.

What to Avoid

Vegetable seed oils like soybean oil, peanut oil and corn oil

Legumes such as peanuts, lentils, soy

Grains like quinoa, rice, wheat, sorghum, oats, millet

Refined sugar

Dairy products

Potatoes

Processed foods

What to eat

Fish and seafood

Green leafy vegetables

Nuts and seeds

Eggs

Grass-fed meat

Herbs and spices

Fruits

Good fats like olive oil, coconut oil

Let us now look at tasty recipes you can try out.

Salad Recipes

Chicken Salad

(Prep + Cook Time: 25 minutes | Servings: 2)

Ingredients:

- 2 tsp. parsley; dried
- 2 chicken breasts; skinless and boneless
- 1/2 tsp. onion powder
- 1/2 cup lemon juice
- 2 tsp. paprika
- A pinch of sea salt
- Black pepper to the taste
- 8 strawberries; sliced
- 1 small red onion; sliced
- 6 cups baby spinach
- 1 avocado; peeled and cut into small chunks
- 1/4 cup extra virgin olive oil
- 1 tbsp. tarragon; chopped
- 2 tbsp. balsamic vinegar

Instructions:

1. Put chicken in a bowl; add lemon juice, parsley, onion powder and paprika and toss to coat.
2. Place chicken on preheated grill over medium high heat, cook for 10 minutes on each side, transfer to a cutting board and slice.
3. In a bowl; mix oil with vinegar, a pinch of sea salt, pepper and tarragon and whisk well.
4. In a salad bowl; mix spinach with onion, avocado and strawberry. Add chicken pieces and the vinaigrette, toss to coat and serve.

4

Nutrition Facts Per Serving: Calories: 230; Fat: 42; Carbs: 13; Fiber: 5; Protein: 30

Lobster Salad

(Prep + Cook Time: 10 minutes | Servings: 2)

Ingredients:

- 1 grapefruit; peeled and chopped
- 1 lb. lobster meat; cooked and chopped
- 1 avocado; pitted, peeled and chopped
- 1 shallot; chopped
- 3 cups mixed greens
- 2 tbsp. grapefruit juice
- 1 tbsp. chives; chopped
- A pinch of sea salt
- Black pepper to the taste
- 4 tbsp. extra virgin olive oil
- 2 tbsp. white wine vinegar
- Some dill; finely chopped for serving

Instructions:

1. In a bowl; mix grapefruit juice with oil, vinegar, chives, shallot, a pinch of sea salt and pepper to the taste and stir very well.
2. Add lobster meat and toss to coat.

3. In a large bowl; mix avocado with greens and grapefruit. Add

   lobster meat and dressing on top, sprinkle dill all over and

   serve.

Nutrition Facts Per Serving: Calories: 180; Fat: 10; Carbs: 6.5; Fiber: 1.4; Sugar: 3.4; Protein: 11.1

Carrot And Cucumber Salad

(Prep + Cook Time: 15 minutes | Servings: 4)

Ingredients:

- 3 carrots; thinly sliced with a spiralizer
- 2 cucumbers; thinly sliced with a spiralizer
- 1 green onion; sliced
- 1 tbsp. sesame seeds
- 2 tbsp. lime juice
- A pinch of sea salt
- 2 tbsp. white wine vinegar
- Black pepper to the taste
- 2 tbsp. extra virgin olive oil

Instructions:

1. In a salad bowl; mix cucumbers with green onion and carrots.

2. In a small bowl; mix vinegar with olive oil, lime juice, a pinch of sea salt and pepper to the taste and stir well. Pour this over salad, toss to coat and keep in the fridge until you serve it.

Nutrition Facts Per Serving: Calories: 60; Fat: 1.7; Carbs: 12; Fiber: 2.5; Protein: 1.3

Paleo Broccoli Salad

(Prep + Cook Time: 12 minutes | Servings: 4)

Ingredients:

- **1/4 cup walnuts; chopped**

- **1/4 cup cranberries**

- **2 bacon slices**

- **4 cups broccoli florets; roughly chopped**

- **1 tsp. lemon juice**

- **1/4 cup olive oil**

Instructions:

1. Heat up a pan over medium high heat, add bacon, cook for 2 minutes, leave aside to cool down and chop.

2. In a salad bowl; mix broccoli with bacon, cranberries, walnuts, lemon juice and olive oil, toss to coat and serve.

Nutrition Facts Per Serving: Calories: 120; Fat: 2; Fiber: 1; Carbs: 5; Protein: 8

Tasty Egg Salad

(Prep + Cook Time: 20 minutes | Servings: 4)

Ingredients:

- 1 avocado; pitted, peeled and chopped
- 1 small red onion; chopped
- 4 eggs
- 1 small red bell pepper; chopped
- 1/4 cup homemade mayonnaise
- A pinch of sea salt
- Black pepper to the taste
- 1 tbsp. lemon juice

Instructions:

1. Put eggs in a pot, add water to cover, place on stove over medium high heat, bring to a boil, reduce heat to low and cook for 10 minutes.
2. Drain eggs, leave them in cold water to cool down, peel, chop them and put in a salad bowl.

3. Add a pinch of sea salt and pepper to the taste, onion, bell

   pepper, avocado, lemon juice and mayo, toss to coat and

   serve right away.

Nutrition Facts Per Serving: Calories: 109; Fat: 4.6; Carbs: 7.5; Fiber: 3.3; Protein: 9

Paleo Beef Salad

(Prep + Cook Time: 20 minutes | Servings: 4)

Ingredients:

- 1 lb. organic beef steak; cut into strips
- 3 cups broccoli; florets separated
- 8 cups baby salad greens
- 1 red onion; sliced
- 1 red bell pepper; sliced

For the vinaigrette:

- 1 tbsp. ginger; minced
- A pinch of sea salt
- Black pepper to the taste
- 1/2 cup extra virgin olive oil
- 2 tbsp. lime juice
- 1 tbsp. rice wine vinegar
- 2 tbsp. shallots; finely chopped

Instructions:

1. In a bowl; mix ginger with oil, lime juice, vinegar, shallots, a pinch of sea salt and pepper to the taste and stir well.
2. Heat up a pan over medium high heat, add 2 tbsp. of vinaigrette, warm up, add broccoli and cook for 3 minutes.
3. Add beef, stir and cook for 4 more minutes and take off heat.
4. In a salad bowl; mix salad greens with onion, bell pepper, broccoli and beef. Add some black pepper, drizzle the rest of the vinaigrette, toss to coat and serve.

Nutrition Facts Per Serving: Calories: 260; Fat: 12; Carbs: 11; Fiber: 4.3; Protein: 32

Brussels Sprouts Salad

(Prep + Cook Time: 20 minutes | Servings: 4)

Ingredients:

- 4 cups Brussels sprouts
- 2 cups red cabbage; shredded
- Black pepper to the taste
- 1 red apple; sliced
- 2 celery stalks; chopped
- 2 tbsp. lemon juice
- 1/4 cup walnuts; chopped
- 1/4 cup homemade mayonnaise
- 4 tbsp. apple cider vinegar

Instructions:

1. In a bowl; mix lemon juice with mayo, vinegar and pepper to the taste and stir very well.

2. In a big bowl; mix Brussels sprouts with cabbage, celery, apple and walnuts. Add salad dressing you've just made, toss to coat and keep in the fridge for 10 minutes before you serve it.

Nutrition Facts Per Serving: Calories: 80; Fat: 1; Carbs: 3; Fiber: 1; Sugar: 1; Protein: 2

Paleo Chicken Salad

(Prep + Cook Time: 10 minutes | Servings: 2)

Ingredients:

- 1 smoked chicken breast; sliced
- 2 handfuls lettuce leaves; torn
- 1 avocado; pitted, peeled and cubed
- 2 eggs; hard-boiled and halved
- A handful walnuts; chopped
- 2 tbsp. flaxseed oil

Instructions:

1. In a salad bowl; mix lettuce with avocado, walnuts and chicken slices and toss.

2. Add eggs and oil, toss gently and serve.

Nutrition Facts Per Serving: Calories: 110; Fat: 0.9; Fiber: 1; Carbs: 4; Protein: 12

Paleo Summer Salad

(Prep + Cook Time: 10 minutes | Servings: 3)

Ingredients:

- 1 lettuce head; chopped
- A handful kale; chopped
- A handful green beans
- A handful walnuts; chopped
- 8 cherry tomatoes; halved
- A handful radishes; chopped
- 1 tbsp. lemon juice
- 8 dates; chopped
- A drizzle of olive oil

Instructions:

1. In a salad bowl; mix lettuce with kale, green beans, walnuts, tomatoes, radishes and dates.

2. In smaller bowl; mix lemon juice with olive oil and whisk

   well. Add this to salad, toss to coat and serve.

Nutrition Facts Per Serving: Calories: 100; Fat: 0; Fiber: 1; Carbs: 1; Protein: 6

Paleo Winter Salad

(Prep + Cook Time: 17 minutes | Servings: 2)

Ingredients:

- 1 red onion; chopped
- 12 Brussels sprouts; sliced
- A pinch of sea salt
- Black pepper to the taste
- 1 tbsp. olive oil
- 1/3 cup pecans; chopped
- 1/4 cup raisins
- 2/3 cup hemp seeds
- 1/2 red apple; cored and chopped

Instructions:

1. Heat up a pan with the oil over medium heat, add onion, stir and cook for a few minutes.

2. Add Brussels sprouts, cook for 4 minutes, take off heat and leave aside to cool down. Add apple pieces, hemp seeds, raisins, a pinch of sea salt, black pepper and pecans, stir salad and serve.

Nutrition Facts Per Serving: Calories: 100; Fat: 0.7; Fiber: 1; Carbs: 3; Protein: 9

Pear Salad With Tasty Dressing

(Prep + Cook Time: 10 minutes | Servings: 4)

Ingredients:

- 1 pear; sliced
- 5 cups lettuce leaves; torn
- 1 small cucumber; chopped
- 1/2 cup cherry tomatoes; cut in halves
- 1/2 cup red grapes; cut in halves
- A pinch of sea salt
- Black pepper to the taste
- 3 tbsp. orange juice
- 1/4 cup extra virgin olive oil
- 1 tbsp. orange zest
- 2 tsp. raw honey
- 1 tbsp. parsley; minced

Instructions:

1. In a bowl; mix orange juice with olive oil, orange zest, honey, a pinch of sea salt, pepper to the taste and parsley and whisk very well.

2. In a salad bowl; mix pear with lettuce, cucumber, tomatoes and grapes. Add salad dressing, toss to coat and serve right away.

Nutrition Facts Per Serving: Calories: 100; Fat: 14; Carbs: 15; Fiber: 1; Protein: 3

Cabbage And Salmon Slaw

(Prep + Cook Time: 18 minutes | Servings: 4)

Ingredients:

- 2 salmon fillets; skin on
- 1½ tsp. coconut aminos
- 1/2 cup mayonnaise
- 1 tsp. lime juice
- 1 tsp. honey
- 1 fennel bulb; sliced
- 1 small red cabbage head; sliced
- A bunch of coriander; chopped
- A pinch of sea salt
- Black pepper to the taste

Instructions:

1. Put water in a pot and bring to a simmer over medium high heat.
2. Place salmon fillets in a vacuum bag, place in water, cook for 8 minutes, leave aside to cool down and cut into medium pieces.
3. Put salmon cubes in a salad bowl; add fennel, cabbage and coriander and toss gently.

4. In another bowl; mix coconut aminos with mayo, lime, honey, salt and pepper and whisk well. Add this to salad, toss to coat well and serve.

Nutrition Facts Per Serving: Calories: 160; Fat: 3; Fiber: 2; Carbs: 5; Protein: 17

Scallops Salad

(Prep + Cook Time: 17 minutes | Servings: 4)

Ingredients:

- 1 lb. bay scallops
- 2 tsp. cayenne pepper
- Black pepper to the taste
- 3 tbsp. lemon juice
- 1 tbsp. homemade mayonnaise
- 1 tsp. mustard
- A pinch of cayenne pepper
- 1/2 cup extra virgin olive oil
- 1 garlic clove; minced
- 2 handfuls mixed greens
- 1 avocado; pitted, peeled and cubed
- 1 red bell pepper; cut into thin strips
- 3 tbsp. melted coconut oil

Instructions:

1. In a salad bowl; mix salad greens with avocado and pepper and leave aside for now.
2. In a bowl; mix lemon juice with mustard, garlic, mayo, pepper and a pinch of cayenne, stir well and leave aside.
3. Add olive oil gradually and whisk very well again.
4. Rinse and pat dry scallops, put them in another bowl; add pepper to the taste and 2 tsp. cayenne and toss to coat.
5. Heat up a pan with the coconut oil over medium high heat, add scallops, cook for 2 minutes on each side and transfer them to the bowl with the veggies. Add mustard dressing you've made, toss to coat and serve.

Nutrition Facts Per Serving: Calories: 235; Fat: 4.1; Carbs: 18; Fiber: 3.3; Protein: 30.7

Summer Salad

(Prep + Cook Time: 15 minutes | Servings: 4)

Ingredients:

- 1 cucumber; chopped
- 4 medium tomatoes; chopped
- 1 red onion; sliced
- 1 green bell pepper; chopped
- 3/4 cup kalamata olives; pitted and chopped
- 1 tbsp. lemon juice
- 1/4 cup extra virgin olive oil
- 1/2 tsp. oregano; dried
- 2 tbsp. red wine vinegar
- Black pepper to the taste

Instructions:

1. In a small bowl; mix lemon juice with oil, oregano, vinegar and pepper to the taste and whisk very well.

2. In a salad bowl; mix tomatoes with bell pepper, onion and cucumber. Add salad dressing, toss to coat and serve with olives on top.

Nutrition Facts Per Serving: Calories: 140; Fat: 9; Carbs: 3; Fiber: 5; Protein: 7

Paleo Summer Salad

(Prep + Cook Time: 10 minutes | Servings: 6)

Ingredients:

- 1 cup blackberries; halved
- 2 cups honeydew; sliced
- 8 oz. prosciutto
- 3 tbsp. chives; chopped
- Juice of 1 lemon
- Zest from 1 lemon
- 1 shallot; chopped
- 2 cup cantaloupe; sliced
- A pinch of sea salt
- Black pepper to the taste

Instructions:

1. In a large salad bowl; mix blackberries with prosciutto, honeydew, cantaloupe, chives, lemon juice and zest, shallot, a pinch of sea salt and black pepper to the taste, toss to coat and serve cold.

Nutrition Facts Per Serving: Calories: 80; Fat: 0.5; Fiber: 1; Carbs: 1; Protein: 3

Chicken Salad

(Prep + Cook Time: 60 minutes | Servings: 4)

Ingredients:

- 2 chicken breasts; skinless and boneless
- 1 pineapple; sliced
- 6 cups mixed salad greens
- 1 red onion; thinly sliced
- 1/4 cup pineapple sauce
- 1/2 cup cherry tomatoes; cut in halves
- A pinch of sea salt
- Black pepper to the taste
- 1/4 cup extra virgin olive oil
- 2 tbsp. apple cider vinegar

For the sauce:

- 1 yellow onion; minced
- 1 garlic clove; minced
- 6 oz. tomato paste
- 1/2 cup apple cider vinegar
- 1/2 cup water
- 1/4 cup ketchup
- 3 tbsp. mustard
- 1 pinch cloves; ground
- A pinch of cinnamon
- A pinch of smoked paprika

Instructions:

1. Heat up a pan over medium high heat, add 1 yellow onion, stir and brown for 3 minutes.
2. Add garlic and cook 1 more minute.
3. Add tomato paste, 1/2 cup vinegar, water, ketchup, mustard, cloves, cinnamon and a pinch of smoked paprika, stir everything well, bring to a boil, reduce heat to medium-low and simmer for 30 minutes.

4. Take sauce off heat, reserve 1 cup and keep the rest in the fridge for another occasion.
5. Season chicken breast with a pinch of sea salt and pepper to the taste, place them on preheated grill over medium high heat, cook for 8 minutes on each side.
6. Brush chicken with 1 cup of the sauce you've just made and cook for 4 more minutes on each side.
7. Transfer chicken to a cutting board, leave aside to cool down, slice and put in a salad bowl.
8. Grill pineapple on medium high heat, transfer to a cutting board as well, cut into small cubes and add to chicken.
9. Also add greens, red onion, grape tomatoes and pepper to the taste.
10. In a small bowl; mix pineapple juice with 2 tbsp. vinegar, 1/4 cup olive oil, a pinch of sea salt and pepper to the taste and stir well. Pour this over chicken salad, toss to coat and serve.

Nutrition Facts Per Serving: Calories: 120; Fat: 16; Carbs: 45; Fiber: 4; Protein: 16

Special Paleo Salad

(Prep + Cook Time: 30 minutes | Servings: 4)

Ingredients:

- 2 red onions; cut into medium wedges
- 1 butternut squash; cut into medium wedges
- 6 cups spinach
- 4 parsnips; cut into medium wedges
- Black pepper to the taste
- 2 tbsp. white wine vinegar
- 1/3 cup nuts; roasted
- 1 tsp. Dijon mustard
- 1/2 tbsp. oregano; dried
- 1 garlic clove; minced
- 6 tbsp. extra virgin olive oil

Instructions:

1. Spread squash, onions and parsnips in a baking dish.
2. Drizzle half of the oil, sprinkle oregano and pepper to the taste, toss to coat, introduce in the oven at 400 °F and bake for 10 minutes.
3. Take veggies out of the oven, turn them and bake for another 10 minutes.
4. In a bowl; mix vinegar with the rest of the oil, garlic, mustard and pepper to the taste and stir very well.

5. Put spinach in a salad bowl; add roasted veggies, pour salad

   dressing, sprinkle nuts, toss to coat and serve warm.

Nutrition Facts Per Serving: Calories: 131; Fat: 5.5; Carbs: 14; Fiber: 4.7; Sugar: 5; Protein: 5.2

Delightful Paleo Salad

(Prep + Cook Time: 50 minutes | Servings: 4)

Ingredients:

- 2 tbsp. ghee
- 1 tbsp. balsamic vinegar
- 1 zucchini; cubed
- 4 bacon strips
- 4 eggs
- 2 lettuce heads; leaves, torn
- 2 cups chicken meat; already cooked and shredded
- 4 cups arugula
- 1 small red onion; finely chopped
- 1/3 cup cranberries
- A pinch of sea salt
- Black pepper to the taste
- A pinch of garlic powder
- 1/3 cup pecans; chopped
- 2 apples; chopped
- 2 tbsp. maple syrup
- 1 tbsp. apple cider vinegar
- 1 tsp. shallot; minced
- 1 tsp. mustard
- 1 tsp. garlic; minced
- 1/4 cup extra virgin olive oil

Instructions:

1. Spread zucchini cubes on a lined baking sheet, sprinkle with a pinch of sea salt, pepper, garlic powder, drizzle balsamic vinegar and add ghee, toss to coat, introduce in the oven at 400 °F and bake for 25 minutes.
2. Meanwhile; put eggs in a pot, add water to cover, bring to a boil over medium high heat, boil for 15 minutes, drain, place in a bowl filled with ice water, leave aside to cool down, peel them, chop and put in a salad bowl.

3. Heat up a pan over medium high heat, add bacon, brown for a few minutes, take off heat, leave to cool down and add to the same bowl with the eggs.
4. Add lettuce leaves, arugula, chicken, onion, pecans, apple pieces, roasted squash cubes and cranberries.

5. In a small bowl; mix maple syrup with apple cider vinegar,

   mustard, garlic, shallot, olive oil and pepper and whisk very

   well. Pour this over salad, toss to coat and serve.

Nutrition Facts Per Serving: Calories: 249; Fat: 10; Carbs: 35; Fiber: 6; Sugar: 2.8; Protein: 5

Paleo Salmon Salad

(Prep + Cook Time: 15 minutes | Servings: 2)

Ingredients:

- 1 lettuce head; chopped
- 2 salmon fillets
- 1 tbsp. olive oil
- 1 tbsp. coconut aminos
- 1 avocado; pitted, peeled and sliced
- 1 cucumber; sliced
- A pinch of sea salt
- Black pepper to the taste

Instructions:

1. Heat up a pan with the oil over medium high heat, add salmon fillets skin side down, cook for 3 minutes, flip and cook for 2 minutes more.

2. In a salad bowl; mix lettuce with cucumber, avocado, a pinch of salt, black pepper and coconut aminos and stir. Flake salmon using a fork, add to salad, drizzle some of the oil from the pan, toss to coat and serve.

Nutrition Facts Per Serving: Calories: 140; Fat: 3; Fiber: 2; Carbs: 6; Protein: 15

Radish Salad

(Prep + Cook Time: 10 minutes | Servings: 4)

Ingredients:

- 8 radishes; sliced
- 1 cucumber; sliced
- 1 apple; chopped
- 1 celery stalk; chopped
- Black pepper to the taste
- 1/4 cup homemade mayonnaise
- 2 tbsp. chives; chopped
- 2 tbsp. apple cider vinegar
- 2 tbsp. lemon juice

Instructions:

1. In a bowl; mix radishes with apple, celery and cucumber.

2. In a small bowl; mix mayo with vinegar, pepper, lemon juice

   and chives and whisk well. Pour this over salad, toss to coat

   and keep in the fridge until you serve it.

Nutritional value: Calories: 50; Fat: 7; Carbs: 3; Fiber: 1; Protein: 1

Awesome Steak Salad

(Prep + Cook Time: 1 hour 15 minutes | Servings: 4)

Ingredients:

- 4 cups lettuce leaves; torn
- 1 lb. steak
- 1 red bell pepper; cut into strips
- 1 cucumber; sliced
- 1/4 cup mint leaves; chopped
- 1/4 cup cilantro; chopped
- 1 tbsp. ginger; grated
- 1/4 cup coconut aminos
- 1 Thai red chili pepper; chopped
- 3 garlic cloves; minced
- Juice from 1 lime
- A pinch of sea salt
- Black pepper to the taste
- Silvered almonds for serving

For the salad dressing:

- 3 tbsp. coconut aminos
- 2 tbsp. melted coconut oil
- 1 tsp. fish sauce
- Zest from 1 lime
- Juice from 1 lime
- 1 Thai red chili pepper; chopped

Instructions:

1. In a bowl; mix garlic with ginger, 1 red chili, juice from 1 lime and 1/4 cup coconut aminos and stir.
2. Add steak, toss to coat, cover bowl and keep in the fridge for 1 hour.
3. In another bowl; mix 2 tbsp. coconut oil with 3 tbsp. coconut aminos, 1 lime chili pepper, fish sauce, zest and juice from 1 lime, stir well and leave aside for now.

4. Place steak on preheated grill over medium high heat, cook for 4 minutes on each side, transfer to a cutting board, leave aside for 4 minutes, slice very thinly and put in a salad bowl.

5. Add lettuce, cucumber, bell pepper, a pinch of sea salt and

    pepper to the taste. Add salad dressing you've made, toss to

    coat, sprinkle cilantro, mint and almonds and serve.

Nutrition Facts Per Serving: Calories: 300; Fat: 10; Carbs: 15; Fiber: 4; Sugar: 4; Protein: 38

Shrimp Salad

(Prep + Cook Time: 30 minutes | Servings: 2)

Ingredients:

- 5 cups mixed greens
- 1/2 cup cherry tomatoes; cut in halves
- 1 lb. shrimp; peeled and deveined
- 1 small red onion; thinly sliced
- 1 avocado; pitted, peeled and chopped
- Black pepper to the taste
- 1/2 tbsp. sweet paprika
- 1/2 tsp. cumin
- 1 tbsp. chili powder
- 1/3 cup cilantro; finely chopped
- 1/2 cup lime juice
- 1/4 cup extra virgin olive oil

Instructions:

1. In a bowl; mix chili powder with cumin, paprika, 1/4 cup lime juice and shrimp, toss to coat and leave aside for 20 minutes.
2. Place shrimps on preheated grill over medium high heat, cook for 4 minutes on each side and transfer to a bowl.
3. In a small bowl; mix cilantro with oil, the rest of the lime juice and pepper to the taste and whisk very well.

4. In a large salad bowl; mix greens with tomatoes, onion, avocado and shrimp. Add salad dressing, toss to coat and serve right away.

Nutrition Facts Per Serving: Calories: 190; Fat: 40; Carbs: 19; Fiber: 3; Protein: 50

Pomegranate Salad

(Prep + Cook Time: 15 minutes | Servings: 4)

Ingredients:

- 1 avocado; pitted, peeled and chopped
- 8 cups mixed salad greens
- 2 tbsp. pine nuts; toasted
- 6 figs; cut into quarters
- 3/4 cup pomegranate seeds
- 4 clementines; peeled and chopped
- 1/4 cup extra virgin olive oil
- 1 tbsp. lemon juice
- 4 tbsp. orange juice
- 2 tbsp. white wine vinegar
- 1 tsp. orange zest
- A pinch of sea salt
- Black pepper to the taste

Instructions:

1. In a salad bowl; mix greens with avocado, figs, clementines, pine nuts and pomegranate seeds.

2. In another bowl; mix orange juice with lemon juice, olive oil, orange zest, vinegar, a pinch of sea salt and pepper to the taste and whisk well. Pour this over salad, toss to coat and serve.

Nutrition Facts Per Serving: Calories: 120; Fat: 6; Carbs: 12; Fiber: 2; Protein: 4.7

Eggplant And Tomato Salad

(Prep + Cook Time: 18 minutes | Servings: 4)

Ingredients:

- 1/2 cup sun-dried tomatoes; sliced
- 1 eggplant; sliced
- 1 green onion; sliced
- Black pepper to the taste
- 4 cups mixed salad greens
- 1 tbsp. mint leaves; finely chopped
- 1 tbsp. oregano; finely chopped
- 1 tbsp. parsley leaves; finely chopped
- 4 tbsp. extra virgin olive oil

For the salad dressing:

- 2 garlic cloves; minced
- 1/4 cup extra virgin olive oil
- 1/2 tbsp. mustard
- 1 tbsp. lemon juice
- 1/2 tsp. smoked paprika
- A pinch of sea salt
- Black pepper to the taste

Instructions:

1. Brush eggplant slices with olive oil, season with black pepper, place them on preheated grill over medium high heat, cook for 3 minutes on each side and transfer them to a salad bowl.
2. Add sun-dried tomatoes, onion, greens, mint, parsley, oregano and pepper to the taste and 4 tbsp. olive oil and toss to coat.

3. In a small bowl; mix 1/4 cup olive oil with garlic, mustard, paprika, lemon juice, salt and pepper to the taste and whisk very well. Pour this over salad, toss to coat gently and serve.

Nutrition Facts Per Serving: Calories: 130; Fat: 27; Carbs: 14; Fiber: 2; Protein: 4

Paleo Kale And Carrots Salad

(Prep + Cook Time: 10 minutes | Servings: 1)

Ingredients:

- 1 carrot; grated
- A handful kale; chopped
- 1 small lettuce head; chopped
- 1 tbsp. tahini paste
- 1 tbsp. olive oil
- A pinch of sea salt
- Black pepper to the taste
- Juice of 1/2 lime
- A pinch of garlic powder

Instructions:

1. In a salad bowl; mix carrots with kale and lettuce leaves.
2. In your blender, mix tahini with a pinch of salt, black pepper, garlic powder, lime juice and oil and pulse well.

3. Pour this over salad, toss to coat well and serve.

Nutrition Facts Per Serving: Calories: 100; Fat: 1; Fiber: 0; Carbs: 0; Protein: 7

Paleo Sashimi Salad

(Prep + Cook Time: 10 minutes | Servings: 2)

Ingredients:

- 1 tsp. balsamic vinegar
- 1/2 tbsp. honey
- 1 mango; peeled and roughly chopped
- 2 handfuls kale; chopped
- 1/2 lb. salmon sashimi; sliced
- 3 tbsp. tamari sauce
- 2 tbsp. olive oil

Instructions:

1. In a bowl; mix tamari with oil, honey and vinegar and whisk well.

2. In a salad bowl; mix kale with mango and sashimi. Add salad dressing, toss to coat and serve.

Nutrition Facts Per Serving: Calories: 140; Fat: 1; Fiber: 2; Carbs: 2; Protein: 16

Potato Salad

(Prep + Cook Time: 45 minutes | Servings: 4)

Ingredients:

- 8 sweet potatoes; chopped
- 1 tbsp. coriander seeds
- 1 tsp. cumin seeds
- 1 red onion; sliced
- 1/2 tbsp. oregano; dried
- A pinch of sea salt
- Black pepper to the taste
- 4 bacon slices; already cooked and crumbled
- 1/2 tsp. chili flakes
- 1/4 cup extra virgin olive oil
- 3 tbsp. parsley; chopped
- 1 tbsp. coconut oil
- 2 tbsp. red wine vinegar

Instructions:

1. Put potatoes in a pot, add water to cover, bring to a boil over medium high heat, cook for 20 minutes, drain water and put them in a bowl.
2. Heat up a pan with the coconut oil over medium high heat, add onions, stir; reduce temperature to low, cook for 10 minutes and transfer them to a bowl
3. Return pan to medium high heat, add cumin seeds and coriander seeds, stir; toast for 2 minutes and add them to the bowl with the onions.

4. Also add chili flakes, oregano, bacon, parsley, olive oil, vinegar, a pinch of sea salt and pepper to the taste and stir everything well. Add potatoes, toss to coat and serve cold.

Nutrition Facts Per Serving: Calories: 142; Fat: 24; Carbs: 47; Fiber: 2; Protein: 10

Paleo Chorizo Salad

(Prep + Cook Time: 30 minutes | Servings: 4)

Ingredients:

- 4 cups arugula
- 1 tbsp. rosemary; chopped
- 2 green onions; chopped
- 2 chorizo sausages; sliced
- 1 tbsp. bacon fat
- 2 garlic cloves; minced
- 4 sweet potatoes; peeled and cubed
- A pinch of sea salt
- Black pepper to the taste

For the salad dressing:

- 2 tsp. mustard
- 2 tbsp. apple vinegar
- 4 tbsp. olive oil
- 1/2 tsp. lemon juice

Instructions:

1. Heat up a pan with the bacon fat over medium heat, add sweet potatoes, stir and cook for 7 minutes.
2. Add a pinch of salt, black pepper, rosemary and garlic, stir and cook for 6 minutes more.
3. Add chorizo slices, stir; cook for 3 minutes, take off heat, cool down and transfer everything to a salad bowl.
4. Add green onions and arugula and stir.

5. In a small bowl; mix olive oil with lemon juice, vinegar, mustard and some black pepper and whisk well. Add this to salad, toss to coat and serve.

Nutrition Facts Per Serving: Calories: 190; Fat: 3; Fiber: 2; Carbs: 5; Protein: 9

Awesome Pork Salad

(Prep + Cook Time: 15 minutes | Servings: 4)

Ingredients:

- 2 lettuce heads; torn
- 2 cups pork; already cooked and shredded
- 1 avocado; pitted, peeled and chopped
- 1 cup cherry tomatoes; cut in halves
- 1 green bell pepper; sliced
- 2 green onions; thinly sliced
- A pinch of sea salt
- Black pepper to the taste
- Juice of 1/2 lime
- 1 tbsp. apple cider vinegar
- 1/4 cup BBQ sauce
- 2 tbsp. extra virgin olive oil

Instructions:

1. In a small bowl; mix oil with lime juice, vinegar, black pepper and BBQ sauce and whisk well.
2. Heat up a pan over medium heat, add pork meat and heat it up.
3. Meanwhile; in a salad bowl; mix lettuce leaves with tomatoes, bell pepper, avocado and green onions. Add pork, drizzle the BBQ dressing, toss to coat and serve.

Nutrition Facts Per Serving: Calories: 322; Fat: 45; Carbs: 23; Fiber: 4; Protein: 36

Seafood Salad

(Prep + Cook Time: 3 hours 10 minutes | Servings: 6)

Ingredients:

- 8 ounces; baby shrimp, already cooked, peeled, deveined and chopped
- 8 oz. crab meat; already cooked
- 2/3 cup homemade mayonnaise
- 2/3 cup yellow onion; chopped
- 2/3 cup celery; chopped
- 2 tbsp. Dijon mustard
- Black pepper to the taste
- 1/4 tsp. onion powder
- 1/2 tsp. garlic powder
- 1 tbsp. hot sauce

Instructions:

1. In a salad bowl; mix shrimp with crab meat, onion and celery.

2. In another bowl; mix mayo with mustard, pepper, onion powder, garlic powder and hot sauce and stir very well. Pour this over seafood salad, toss to coat and keep in the fridge for 3 hours before you serve it.

Nutrition Facts Per Serving: Calories: 240; Fat: 22; Carbs: 3.3; Fiber: 0.6; Protein: 24

Paleo Taco Salad

(Prep + Cook Time: 25 minutes | Servings: 4)

Ingredients:

- 1 tbsp. chili powder
- 1 tsp. onion powder
- 1/2 tsp. garlic powder
- 1 tsp. cumin; ground
- 2 tsp. paprika
- 3 tbsp. olive oil
- A pinch of cayenne pepper
- 1 lb. beef; ground
- 3 cups cilantro; chopped
- Juice from 1 lime
- A pinch of sea salt
- Black pepper to the taste
- 1 romaine lettuce head; chopped
- 1 avocado; pitted, peeled and chopped
- 1 small red onion; chopped
- Some black olives; pitted and chopped
- 1 red bell pepper; chopped
- 1/2 cup Pico de gallo

Instructions:

1. In a bowl; mix chili powder with paprika, onion and garlic powder, 1/2 tsp. cumin, cayenne and some black pepper and stir.
2. Heat up a pan with 1 tbsp. oil over medium heat, add beef, stir and cook for 7 minutes.
3. Add spice mix, stir and cook until meat is done.
4. Meanwhile; in your food processor, blend 1 cup cilantro with lime juice, 1/2 tsp. cumin, a pinch of salt, black pepper to the taste and 2 tbsp. oil and pulse really well.

5. In a salad bowl; mix lettuce leaves with avocado, 2 cups cilantro, onion, bell pepper, olives and Pico de gallo and stir. Divide this between plates, top with beef and drizzle the salad dressing on top.

Nutrition Facts Per Serving: Calories: 190; Fat: 3; Fiber: 2; Carbs: 5; Protein: 12

Green Apple And Shrimp Salad

(Prep + Cook Time: 10 minutes | Servings: 3)

Ingredients:

- 1 green apple; cored and chopped
- 2 cups shrimp; peeled, deveined, cooked and chopped
- 3 eggs; hard-boiled, peeled and chopped
- 1 small red onion; chopped
- 1/4 cup Dijon mustard
- 4 celery stalks; chopped
- 1 tbsp. olive oil
- 2 tbsp. vinegar
- 1/2 tsp. thyme; chopped
- 1/2 tsp. parsley; chopped
- 1/2 tsp. basil; chopped
- A pinch of sea salt
- Black pepper to the taste

Instructions:

1. In a big salad bowl; mix apple pieces with shrimp, eggs, onion and celery and stir.

2. In another bowl; mix mustard with oil, vinegar, thyme, parsley, basil, a pinch of salt and black pepper and whisk well. Add this to your salad, toss well and serve.

Nutritional value: Calories: 110; Fat: 2; Fiber: 4; Carbs: 7; Protein: 15

Sweet Potato Salad

(Prep + Cook Time: 40 minutes | Servings: 4)

Ingredients:

- 3 sweet potatoes; cubed
- 2 tbsp. coconut oil
- 4 garlic cloves; minced
- 1/2 lb. bacon; chopped
- Juice from 1 lime
- A pinch of sea salt
- Black pepper to the taste
- 2 tbsp. balsamic vinegar
- 2 tbsp. olive oil
- A handful dill; chopped
- 2 green onions; chopped
- A pinch of cinnamon; ground
- A pinch of red pepper flakes

Instructions:

1. Arrange bacon and sweet potatoes on a lined bacon sheet, add garlic and coconut oil, toss well, place in the oven at 375 °F and bake for 30 minutes.
2. Meanwhile; in a bowl, mix vinegar with lime juice, olive oil, green onions, pepper flakes, dill, a pinch of sea salt, black pepper and cinnamon and stir well.

3. Transfer bacon and sweet potatoes to a salad bowl; add salad dressing, toss well and serve.

Nutrition Facts Per Serving: Calories: 170; Fat: 3; Fiber: 2; Carbs: 5; Protein: 12

Broccoli And Carrots Salad

(Prep + Cook Time: 10 minutes | Servings: 2)

Ingredients:

- 3 carrots; sliced
- 1 cup broccoli; chopped
- 1/3 cup mushrooms; sliced
- 2 tbsp. walnuts; chopped
- 3 tbsp. red onion; chopped
- 3 tbsp. black olives; pitted and chopped
- A pinch of sea salt
- Black pepper to the taste
- 1 tsp. mustard
- 3 tbsp. olive oil
- 1½ tbsp. red vinegar

Instructions:

1. In a salad bowl; mix carrots with olives, onion, walnuts, mushrooms and broccoli.

2. In a small bowl; mix oil with vinegar, mustard, salt and pepper and whisk well. Add this to salad, toss to coat and serve.

Nutrition Facts Per Serving: Calories: 140; Fat: 1; Fiber: 3; Carbs: 4; Protein: 15

Paleo Rich Salad

(Prep + Cook Time: 10 minutes | Servings: 1)

Ingredients:

- 1 chicken breast; cooked and sliced
- 1 medium lettuce head; chopped
- 1 sweet potato; boiled and cubed
- 1 tbsp. pumpkin seeds
- 6 black olives; pitted and chopped
- 1 tbsp. olive oil
- 1 tbsp. balsamic vinegar

Instructions:

1. In a salad bowl; mix chicken breast slices with lettuce, sweet

   potato, pumpkin seeds, olives, olive oil and balsamic vinegar,

   stir well and serve right away.

Nutrition Facts Per Serving: Calories: 130; Fat: 2; Fiber: 1; Carbs: 4; Protein: 8

Quick Paleo Salad

(Prep + Cook Time: 10 minutes | Servings: 4)

Ingredients:

For the salad dressing:

- 1 tbsp. basil; chopped
- 1 tsp. rosemary ; chopped
- 1/2 cup avocado mayonnaise
- 1 garlic clove; minced
- A pinch of sea salt
- Black pepper to the taste
- 1 tsp. lemon juice

For the salad:

- 6 baby lettuce heads; chopped
- 1 cup cherry tomatoes; halved
- 1/2 lb. bacon; cooked and chopped
- 2 green onions; chopped

Instructions:

1. In a bowl; mix basil with rosemary, mayo, garlic, lemon juice, a pinch of salt and black pepper and whisk well.

2. In a salad bowl; mix lettuce with tomatoes, green onions and

   bacon. Add salad dressing, toss to coat and serve.

Nutrition Facts Per Serving: Calories: 140; Fat: 3; Fiber: 2; Carbs: 4; Protein: 15

Red Cabbage Salad

(Prep + Cook Time: 25 minutes | Servings: 4)

Ingredients:

- 1 purple cabbage head; cut into thin strips
- 4 prosciutto slices
- 1 red onion; thinly sliced
- 1 green apple; cored and chopped
- 1/2 cup pecans; toasted
- A handful watercress
- 1/2 cup olive oil
- 1 garlic clove; minced
- 1/4 cup balsamic vinegar
- 1 tsp. honey
- 1/2 tsp. mustard
- A pinch of sea salt
- Black pepper to the taste

Instructions:

1. Place prosciutto slices on a lined baking sheet, place in the oven at 350 °F and cook for 15 minutes.
2. Leave prosciutto to cool down and chop it.
3. In a salad bowl mix cabbage with prosciutto, onion, apple pieces, watercress and pecans and toss.

4. In another bowl; mix olive oil with honey, vinegar, garlic, mustard, a pinch of salt and black pepper and whisk well.

   Drizzle this over your salad and serve.

Nutrition Facts Per Serving: Calories: 110; Fat: 0.8; Fiber: 1; Carbs: 2; Protein: 7

Russian Salad

Ingredients:

- 1/2 cup walnuts; chopped
- 1/4 cup Paleo mayo anise
- 1½ lbs. beets; roasted, peeled and grated
- 1/2 cup raisins
- 2 garlic cloves; minced
- 1/4 cup parsley; chopped
- A pinch of sea salt
- Black pepper to the taste

Instructions:

1. In a salad bowl; mix grated beets with walnuts, raisins, garlic, parsley, salt and pepper and stir.

2. Add mayo, stir well and serve cold.

Nutrition Facts Per Serving: Calories: 150; Fat: 4; Fiber: 3; Carbs: 3; Protein: 8

Simple Cucumber Salad

(Prep + Cook Time: 10 minutes | Servings: 4)

Ingredients:

- 1 zucchini; cut with a spiralizer
- 3 big cucumbers; cut with a spiralizer
- 2 garlic cloves; minced
- 1½ tbsp. balsamic vinegar
- 1/4 tsp. ginger; grated
- A pinch of sea salt
- Black pepper to the taste
- 2 tsp. sesame oil
- 1 small red jalapeno pepper; chopped
- 5 mint leaves; chopped

Instructions:

1. In a salad bowl; mix zucchini noodles with cucumber ones, garlic, ginger, salt and pepper and stir.

2. Add vinegar, oil, jalapeno and mint, toss to coat and serve right away.

Nutrition Facts Per Serving: Calories: 90; Fat: 0; Fiber: 1; Carbs: 1; Protein: 5

Shrimp Cobb Salad

(Prep + Cook Time: 14 minutes | Servings: 4)

Ingredients:

- 4 bacon strips; cooked and chopped
- 1 tbsp. bacon fat
- 1 lb. shrimp; peeled and deveined
- 1 tsp. garlic powder
- A pinch of sea salt
- Black pepper to the taste
- 6 cups romaine lettuce leaves; chopped
- 4 eggs; hard-boiled, peeled and chopped
- 1-pint cherry tomatoes; halved
- 1 avocado; pitted, peeled and chopped

For the vinaigrette:

- 1 garlic clove, minced
- 2 tbsp. Paleo mayonnaise
- 2 tbsp. vinegar
- 3 tbsp. avocado oil

Instructions:

1. In a bowl mix garlic with mayo, vinegar and avocado oil, whisk well and leave aside for now.
2. Heat up a pan with the bacon fat over medium high heat, add shrimp, season with a pinch of salt, some black pepper and garlic powder, cook for 2 minutes, flip, cook for 2 minutes more and transfer them to a salad bowl.

3. Add tomatoes, avocado pieces, lettuce leaves, bacon and egg pieces and stir.Add the vinaigrette you've made earlier, toss to coat and serve.

Nutrition Facts Per Serving: Calories: 150; Fat: 1; Fiber: 2; Carbs: 6; Protein: 10

Delicious Paleo Dinner Salad

(Prep + Cook Time: 10 minutes | Servings: 2)

Ingredients:

- 1½ tbsp. vinegar
- 3 tbsp. olive oil
- 1 tsp. thyme; dried
- 2 tbsp. macadamia nuts; chopped
- A pinch of sea salt
- Black pepper to the taste
- 3/4 cup chicken; cooked and shredded
- 3 tbsp. onion; chopped
- 1/4 cup carrot; grated
- 4 radishes; chopped
- 1/2 cup red cabbage; shredded
- 1/2 cup green cabbage; shredded

Instructions:

1. In a salad bowl; mix chicken with macadamia nuts, carrot, onion, radishes, green and red cabbage.

2. In a bowl; mix vinegar with oil, a pinch of salt, black pepper and thyme and whisk well. Add this to salad, toss to coat and serve.

Nutrition Facts Per Serving: Calories: 120; Fat: 2; Fiber: 3; Carbs: 4; Protein: 12

Paleo Tomato Salad

(Prep + Cook Time: 10 minutes | Servings: 4)

Ingredients:

- 1 bunch kale; chopped
- 12 cherry tomatoes; halved
- 2 handful green beans
- 3 tbsp. Paleo mayonnaise
- 1 tsp. mustard

Instructions:

1. In a salad bowl; mix tomatoes with green beans and kale.

2. In a small bowl; mix mayo with mustard and whisk well. Add

    this to salad, toss to coat and serve.

Nutrition Facts Per Serving: Calories: 110; Fat: 2; Fiber: 1; Carbs: 3; Protein: 5

Tomato And Chicken Salad

(Prep + Cook Time: 10 minutes | Servings: 6)

Ingredients:

- 3 tbsp. oil
- 4 tbsp. balsamic vinegar
- A pinch of sea salt
- Black pepper to the taste
- 3 cups chicken; cooked and shredded
- 2 lbs. cherry tomatoes; halved
- 1/2 cup red onion; chopped
- 2 tbsp. basil; chopped
- 2 tbsp. chives; chopped
- 2 tbsp. parsley; chopped
- 1 tbsp. thyme; chopped

Instructions:

1. In a salad bowl; mix chicken with tomatoes, onion, basil, chives, parsley and thyme and stir.

2. In a small bowl; mix oil with vinegar, a pinch of salt and black pepper and whisk well. Add this to salad, toss to coat and serve.

Nutrition Facts Per Serving: Calories: 140; Fat: 3; Fiber: 1; Carbs: 2; Protein: 16

Watermelon Salad

(Prep + Cook Time: 1 hour 10 minutes | Servings: 4)

Ingredients:

- 8 cups mixed salad greens
- 4 cups watermelon; cubed
- 1/4 cup mayonnaise
- 1½ tbsp. honey
- 2 tsp. balsamic vinegar
- 1 tsp. poppy seeds
- A pinch of sea salt
- Black pepper to the taste

Instructions:

1. In a salad bowl; mix salad greens with watermelon cubes.

2. In another bowl; mix mayo with honey, vinegar and poppy seeds, whisk well and keep in the fridge for 1 hour. Drizzle this over salad, season with a pinch of salt and black pepper to the taste, toss to coat well and serve.

Nutrition Facts Per Serving: Calories: 120; Fat: 0.5; Fiber: 1; Carbs: 0; Protein: 6

Avocado Salad

(Prep + Cook Time: 10 minutes | Servings: 2)

Ingredients:

- Juice of 1 lemon
- 1 avocado; pitted, peeled and chopped
- 1 tbsp. onion; chopped
- 5 oz. canned wild tuna; flaked
- Black pepper to the taste

Instructions:

1. In a salad bowl; mix avocado with onion, tuna, black pepper

    and lemon juice, toss well and serve.

Nutrition Facts Per Serving: Calories: 90; Fat: 0; Fiber: 1; Carbs: 0; Protein: 12

Kale And Avocado Salad

(Prep + Cook Time: 10 minutes | Servings: 4)

Ingredients:

- 2 tbsp. olive oil
- 1 tsp. maple syrup
- 3 tbsp. lemon juice
- 2 basil leaves; chopped
- 1 garlic clove; minced
- 1 avocado; pitted, peeled and chopped
- 1 bunch kale; chopped
- 1 cup grapes; seedless and halved
- 1/4 cup pumpkin seeds
- 1/3 cup red onion; chopped

Instructions:

1. In a salad bowl; mix kale with avocado, grapes, pumpkin seeds and onion and stir;

2. In another bowl; mix oil with maple syrup, lemon juice, basil and garlic and whisk well. Add this to salad, toss to coat and serve.

Nutrition Facts Per Serving: Calories: 120; Fat: 1; Fiber: 1; Carbs: 2; Protein: 11

Fresh Paleo Salad

(Prep + Cook Time: 10 minutes | Servings: 4)

Ingredients:

- 2 cup red cabbage; chopped
- 4 cups Brussels sprouts; shredded
- 2 tbsp. lemon juice
- 4 tbsp. balsamic vinegar
- 1/4 cup Paleo mayonnaise
- 1 red apple; cored and chopped
- 2 celery sticks; chopped
- 1/4 cup walnuts; chopped
- A pinch of sea salt
- Black pepper to the taste

Instructions:

1. In a salad bowl; mix cabbage with Brussels sprouts, apple, celery and walnuts.

2. In another bowl; mix lemon juice with vinegar, a pinch of salt, black pepper and mayo and whisk well. Add this to salad, toss to coat and serve.

Nutrition Facts Per Serving: Calories: 90; Fat: 0; Fiber: 1; Carbs: 1; Protein: 7

Hearty Paleo Chicken Salad

(Prep + Cook Time: 1 hour 10 minutes | Servings: 6)

Ingredients:

- 1 rotisserie chicken; chopped
- 1 apple; cored and chopped
- 1/4 cup cranberries; dried
- 1/4 cup chives; chopped
- 1/4 cup red onion; chopped
- 1 celery stalk; chopped
- A pinch of sea salt
- Black pepper to the taste
- 2 cups mayonnaise
- 8 handfuls arugula
- 7 avocados; pitted, peeled and chopped

For the vinaigrette:

- 1 garlic clove, minced
- 1/2 cup olive oil
- 1 tsp. mustard
- 3 tbsp. lemon juice
- Black pepper to the taste

Instructions:

1. In a salad bowl; mix chicken meat with apple, cranberries, chives, onion, celery, arugula, avocados, mayo, a pinch of salt and black pepper to the taste and toss well.

2. In a small bowl; mix oil with garlic, mustard, black pepper and lemon juice and whisk well. Add this to salad, toss again well and leave aside at room temperature for 1 hour before serving.

Nutrition Facts Per Serving: Calories: 180; Fat: 3; Fiber: 3; Carbs: 6; Protein: 20

Swiss Chard Salad

(Prep + Cook Time: 13 minutes | Servings: 4)

Ingredients:

- 1 garlic clove; minced
- 1 shallot; chopped
- 1 tbsp. rosemary; chopped
- A pinch of sea salt
- Black pepper to the taste
- 2 tbsp. avocado oil
- 1 bunch Swiss chard; sliced
- 1½ cup walnuts; halved
- 1 tbsp. vinegar
- 1 tbsp. lemon juice

Instructions:

1. Heat up a pan with the oil over medium high heat, add garlic, rosemary, shallot, a pinch of salt and black pepper, stir and cook for 3 minutes.

2. Add walnuts, stir; reduce heat and cook for a few seconds more. In a salad bowl; mix Swiss chard with vinegar, lemon juice and shallots mix and toss to coat.

Nutrition Facts Per Serving: Calories: 195; Fat: 2; Fiber: 2; Carbs: 4; Protein: 10

Cuban Radish Salad

(Prep + Cook Time: 10 minutes | Servings: 4)

Ingredients:

- 6 radishes; sliced
- 1 romaine lettuce head; chopped
- 1 avocado; pitted, peeled and chopped
- 2 tomatoes; roughly chopped
- 1 red onion; chopped

For the salad dressing:

- 1/4 cup apple cider vinegar
- 1/2 cup olive oil
- 1/4 cup lime juice
- 3 garlic cloves; minced
- A pinch of sea salt
- Black pepper to the taste

Instructions:

1. In a salad bowl; mix radishes with lettuce leaves, avocado, onion and tomatoes and stir.

2. In another bowl; mix vinegar with oil, lime juice, garlic, a pinch of salt and black pepper and whisk well. Add this to salad, toss to coat and serve.

Nutrition Facts Per Serving: Calories: 100; Fat: 0.6; Fiber: 1; Carbs: 2; Protein: 4

Paleo Steak Salad

(Prep + Cook Time: 10 minutes | Servings: 4)

Ingredients:

- 6 cups romaine lettuce; chopped
- 1 red onion; chopped
- 1 yellow bell pepper; chopped
- 1 red bell pepper; chopped
- A pinch of sea salt
- Black pepper to the taste
- 1 cucumber; sliced
- 1/2 cup kalamata olives; pitted and sliced
- 1/4 cup parsley; chopped
- 3/4 lb. flank steak; cooked and sliced
- 1 tbsp. olive oil

Instructions:

1. In a salad bowl; mix lettuce with onion, yellow bell pepper, red bell pepper, cucumber, olives, parsley and steak slices and toss well.

2. Add a pinch of salt, black pepper and the oil, toss to coat well

   and serve.

Nutrition Facts Per Serving: Calories: 150; Fat: 3; Fiber: 2; Carbs: 3; Protein: 10

Autumn Salad

(Prep + Cook Time: 14 minutes | Servings: 4)

Ingredients:

For the salad dressing:

- 1 tbsp. parsley; chopped
- 1/3 cup cashew butter
- 1 tbsp. sesame seeds
- 1/2 cup green onion; chopped
- 2 tbsp. tamari sauce
- 2 tbsp. lemon juice
- 2 tbsp. vinegar
- A pinch of sea salt
- Black pepper to the taste
- 2 garlic cloves; minced
- 1/3 cup coconut milk
- 1/4 cup avocado oil

For the salad:

- 2 tbsp. water
- 3 sweet potatoes; cut with a spiralizer
- 1 tbsp. parsley; chopped

Instructions:

1. In your blender, mix cashew butter with 1 tbsp. parsley, green onion, sesame seeds, vinegar, tamari sauce, lemon juice, garlic, coconut milk, a pinch of salt and black pepper and pulse really well.
2. Add the oil gradually and blend again well.
3. Put sweet potato noodles in a bowl; add the water, place in your microwave and steam at High for 4 minutes.

4. Drain potato noodles, transfer to a bowl and add 1 tbsp.

   parsley. Add dressing, toss to coat and serve.

Nutrition Facts Per Serving: Calories: 300; Fat: 4; Fiber: 4; Carbs: 10; Protein: 6

Grilled Shrimp Salad

(Prep + Cook Time: 1 hour 8 minutes | Servings: 4)

Ingredients:

- 1/4 cup ghee; melted
- 1/2 tsp. dill; dried
- 1/4 tsp. smoked paprika
- A pinch of sea salt
- Black pepper to the taste
- 4 bacon slices; cooked and crumbled
- 12 oz. shrimp; peeled and deveined
- 4 cups mixed salad greens
- 1 avocado; pitted, peeled and chopped
- A handful cherry tomatoes; halved
- 2 tbsp. scallions; chopped

Instructions:

1. In a bowl; mix ghee with a pinch of salt, black pepper, dill and paprika and stir well. Put shrimp in a bowl; add half of the ghee mix over them toss well and leave aside in the fridge for 1 hour.
2. Heat up a pan over medium high heat, add shrimp, cook for 3 minutes on each side and transfer to a bowl.

3. Add the rest of the ghee mix, bacon, mixed greens, avocado, tomatoes and scallions, toss everything well and serve.

Nutrition Facts Per Serving: Calories: 200; Fat: 3; Fiber: 5; Carbs: 7; Protein: 15

Chicken Salad And Raspberry Dressing

(Prep + Cook Time: 20 minutes | Servings: 4)

Ingredients:

For the salad dressing:

- 1 tbsp. raspberry vinegar
- 1 shallot; chopped
- 6 oz. raspberries
- 2/3 cup walnuts; chopped
- A pinch of sea salt
- Black pepper to the taste
- 1/4 cup olive oil

For the salad:

- 1/2 tsp. garlic powder
- 1 tbsp. olive oil
- 1/4 tsp. smoked paprika
- 1/4 tsp. turmeric
- Black pepper to the taste
- 2 chicken breast halves
- 1 tbsp. ghee
- 5 oz. baby arugula
- 1 yellow bell pepper; chopped
- 8 oz. strawberries; halved
- 1 avocado; pitted, peeled and chopped
- 1/4 red cabbage; shredded
- 1 cup blueberries

Instructions:

1. Put walnuts in your food processor, blend well and transfer to a bowl.
2. Add vinegar, raspberries, shallots, oil, a pinch of salt and black pepper, whisk well and leave aside for now.
3. Meanwhile; in a bowl, mix 1 tbsp. oil with garlic powder, black pepper, paprika and turmeric and whisk well.

4. Brush chicken breast halves with this mix, place them on your grill after you've greased it with the ghee and cook them over medium high heat for 4 minutes on each side.
5. Transfer chicken to a cutting board, leave them to cool down a bit, slice and transfer them to a salad bowl.

6. Add strawberries, avocado, cabbage, blueberries, bell pepper and arugula. Add salad dressing you've made at the beginning, toss to coat and serve.

Nutrition Facts Per Serving: Calories: 150; Fat: 3; Fiber: 2; Carbs: 5; Protein: 18

Cucumber And Tomato Salad

(Prep + Cook Time: 10 minutes | Servings: 4)

Ingredients:

- 2 tbsp. red vinegar
- 3 tbsp. olive oil
- 1 tsp. oregano; chopped
- 1½ lbs. cucumber; sliced
- 1 cup mixed colored tomatoes; halved
- 2 tbsp. mint; chopped
- 1/2 cup red onion; chopped
- 2 tbsp. parsley; chopped
- 2 tbsp. dill; chopped
- A pinch of sea salt
- Black pepper to the taste

Instructions:

1. In a bowl; mix cucumber with tomatoes, onion, mint, parsley, oregano, dill, salt and pepper and stir.

2. Add vinegar and oil, toss to coat and serve.

Nutrition Facts Per Serving: Calories: 90; Fat: 0; Fiber: 1; Carbs: 0; Protein: 7

Salmon And Strawberry Salad

(Prep + Cook Time: 18 minutes | Servings: 4)

Ingredients:

- 1 lb. salmon fillet
- 2 tbsp. olive oil
- 1/4 tsp. coriander; ground
- 1/2 tsp. cumin; ground
- 1 tsp. chili powder
- 1/4 tsp. paprika
- A pinch of sea salt
- Black pepper to the taste
- 6 strawberries; chopped
- 1/4 cup red onion; chopped
- 1 jalapeno; chopped
- Juice from 1 lime
- 1 garlic clove; minced
- 5 oz. baby arugula
- 1/2 avocado; pitted, peeled and chopped
- 3 radishes; chopped

For the vinaigrette:

- 1/4 cup balsamic vinegar
- 1/3 cup olive oil
- 1/2 tsp. lemon zest
- 3 strawberries; chopped
- 1 tbsp. lemon juice
- 1½ tbsp. maple syrup
- 1½ tbsp. mustard

Instructions:

1. chili powder, paprika, a pinch of salt and black pepper to the taste and whisk well.
2. Brush salmon with this mix, place on preheated grill over medium high heat, cook for 6 minutes skin side down, flip, cook for 2 minutes more, transfer to a cutting board, leave

aside to cool down, cut into medium pieces and transfer to a bowl.

3. Add radishes, avocado, 6 strawberries, garlic, arugula, red onion, jalapeno and lime juice and toss gently.
4. In another bowl; mix 1/3 cup oil with 3 strawberries, vinegar, lemon zest, 1 tbsp. lemon juice, maple syrup and mustard and whisk very well.

5. Add this to salad, toss to coat and serve. In a bowl; mix 2

tbsp. oil with coriander, cumin,

Nutrition Facts Per Serving: Calories: 120; Fat: 2; Fiber: 2; Carbs: 4; Protein: 10

Beetroot Salad

(Prep + Cook Time: 35 minutes | Servings: 2)

Ingredients:

- 2 tsp. oregano; dried
- 2 garlic cloves; minced
- 4 chicken thighs; skin on
- Juice of 1/2 lemon
- A pinch of sea salt
- Black pepper to the taste
- 2 tbsp. coconut oil
- 2 tbsp. olive oil

For the pumpkin:

- 1/2 butternut squash; chopped
- 1½ tsp. fennel seeds
- 1 tbsp. olive oil

For the beetroot:

- 1 tbsp. vinegar
- 2 beetroots; cooked, peeled and cut into medium pieces
- 1/3 cup walnuts; chopped
- 1/4 tsp. cinnamon powder
- 1 tbsp. maple syrup

For the salad dressing:

- 1/2 tsp. maple syrup
- 2 tbsp. olive oil
- 1 tbsp. vinegar
- 1/2 tsp. mustard
- 3 cups salad leaves; torn
- A pinch of sea salt
- Black pepper to the taste

Instructions:

1. In a bowl; mix chicken thighs with 2 garlic cloves, oregano juice from 1/2 lemon, 2 tbsp. oil, a pinch of salt and black

pepper, stir; leave aside for 10 minutes and discard marinade.
2. Heat up a pan with the coconut oil over medium high heat, add chicken pieces, cook for 5 minutes on each side, transfer to a cutting board, leave aside to cool down, shred and put in a bowl.
3. In a bowl; mix butternut squash with fennel seeds, a pinch of salt, some black pepper and 1 tbsp. oil, toss well, spread on a lined baking sheet, place in the oven at 360 °F for 20 minutes.
4. Leave butternut squash pieces to cool down and add them to the bowl with the chicken.
5. In a bowl; mix beetroots with 1 tbsp. vinegar and black pepper to the taste, stir well and add to chicken salad as well.
6. Heat up a pan over medium high heat, add walnuts, maple syrup and cinnamon, stir; toast for a few minutes, take off heat, cool down and add to salad bowl.

7. In a small bowl; mix 2 tbsp. oil with1 tbsp. vinegar, 1/2 tsp.

maple syrup, mustard, a pinch of salt and some black pepper

and whisk well. Add salad leaves to the salad bowl; add salad

dressing, toss to coat well and serve.

Nutrition Facts Per Serving: Calories: 160; Fat: 3; Fiber: 4; Carbs: 5; Protein: 20

Radish And Eggs Salad

(Prep + Cook Time: 20 minutes | Servings: 2)

Ingredients:

- 8 radishes; sliced
- 2 eggs
- 1/2 cup green onions; chopped
- 1 tbsp. mayonnaise
- 1/2 tsp. mustard
- 1 tbsp. lemon juice
- A pinch of sea salt
- Black pepper to the taste
- A few lettuce leaves; chopped

Instructions:

1. Put water in a pot, add eggs, bring to a boil over medium high heat, cook for 10 minutes, transfer eggs to a bowl filled with ice water, leave them to cool down, peel and chop them.

2. In a salad bowl; mix lettuce leaves with chopped eggs, green onions and radishes. Add mustard, mayo, lemon juice, a pinch of salt and black pepper, toss to coat well and serve.

Nutrition Facts Per Serving: Calories: 110; Fat: 1; Fiber: 2; Carbs: 4; Protein: 10

Shrimp And Radish Salad

(Prep + Cook Time: 14 minutes | Servings: 4)

Ingredients:

- 2 lbs. shrimp; deveined
- A pinch of sea salt
- Black pepper to the taste
- 2 tbsp. olive oil
- 4 oz. watermelon radish; thinly sliced
- 4 oz. radishes; sliced
- 1/2 cup fennel bulb; chopped
- 4 green onions; chopped
- 1 tsp. maple syrup
- 2 tbsp. lemon juice
- 1/4 cup mint; chopped
- 2 tbsp. mayonnaise

Instructions:

1. Heat up a pan with the oil over medium high heat, add shrimp, season with a pinch of salt and some black pepper, cook for 2 minutes on each side and transfer them to a salad bowl.
2. Add watermelon radish, radishes, fennel and onions and stir gently.

3. In a small bowl; mix maple syrup with lemon juice, mint and mayo and whisk well. Add this to salad, toss to coat well and serve.

Nutrition Facts Per Serving: Calories: 170; Fat: 3; Fiber: 3; Carbs: 6; Protein: 10

Figs And Cabbage Salad

(Prep + Cook Time: 16 minutes | Servings: 4)

Ingredients:

- 1 red cabbage head; shredded
- 2 tbsp. olive oil
- A pinch of sea salt
- Black pepper to the taste
- 1/4 cup balsamic vinegar
- 1/2 tsp. oregano; dried
- 1 yellow onion; chopped
- 1 tbsp. maple syrup
- 2 figs; cut into quarters
- A handful oregano; chopped

Instructions:

1. In a bowl mix cabbage with a pinch of salt and some black pepper, stir well and leave aside.
2. Heat up a pan with half of the oil over medium heat, add onion, stir and cook for 4 minutes.
3. Add dried oregano and vinegar, stir; cook for 5 minutes and take off heat. Add maple syrup, some black pepper and stir well.

4. In a salad bowl; mix squeezed cabbage with onions mix, figs and the rest of the oil, toss to coat and serve with fresh oregano on top.

Nutrition Facts Per Serving: Calories: 140; Fat: 2; Fiber: 2; Carbs: 4; Protein: 9

Vegetable Recipes

Veggies And Fish Mix

(Prep + Cook Time: 42 minutes | Servings: 4)

Ingredients:

- 1 cup hot water
- 1 tbsp. maple syrup
- 2 tbsp. olive oil
- 1 eggplant; chopped
- 3 cups cherry tomatoes; halved
- 1 tsp. Paleo Tabasco sauce
- 1 lb. tuna; cubed
- 1 tsp. balsamic vinegar
- 1/2 cup basil; chopped
- Black pepper to the taste
- A pinch of sea salt

Instructions:

1. In a bowl; mix eggplant pieces with a pinch of salt and black pepper and stir.
2. Heat up a pan with 1 tbsp. oil over medium heat, add eggplant, cook for 6 minutes stirring often and transfer to a bowl.
3. Heat up the pan again with the rest of the oil over medium heat, add tomatoes, cover pan and cook for 6 minutes shaking the pan from time to time.
4. Return eggplant pieces to the pan, add maple syrup, vinegar and hot water, stir; cover and cook for 10 minutes.

5. Add tuna and Tabasco sauce, stir; cover pan again, reduce heat to medium-low and simmer for 10 minutes more.

Sprinkle basil on top, divide veggies and tuna mix between

plates and serve.

Nutrition Facts Per Serving: Calories: 120; Fat: 1; Fiber: 2; Carbs: 5; Protein: 12

Veggies Dish With Tasty Sauce

(Prep + Cook Time: 35 minutes | Servings: 4)

Ingredients:

- 2 carrots; chopped
- 8 mushrooms; sliced
- 4 zucchinis; cut in thin noodles
- 2 cups spinach; torn
- 2 yellow squash; halved and sliced
- 1 tbsp. coconut oil
- 1 cup coconut milk
- Juice of 1 lemon
- A pinch of sea salt
- Black pepper to the taste

For the pesto:

- 1/2 cup extra virgin olive oil
- 2 cups basil
- 1/3 cup pine nuts
- 3 garlic clove; chopped
- A pinch of sea salt
- Black pepper to the taste

Instructions:

1. In your food processor, mix basil with nuts and garlic and pulse well.
2. Add oil, a pinch of salt and pepper, pulse well again, transfer to a bowl and leave aside.

3. Steam carrots, squash, zucchini and mushrooms in a bamboo steamer for 8 minutes, transfer them to a colander, season with a pinch of sea salt and pepper, leave aside for 10 minutes, pat dry them and put in a bowl.
4. Heat up a pan with the oil over medium high heat, add half of the coconut milk, salt and pepper and bring to a boil stirring all the time.
5. Add the pesto you've made, lemon juice and the rest of the coconut milk and stir again.

6. Add steamed veggies, stir and cook for 2 minutes. Add spinach, more salt and pepper if needed, stir; cook for 2 minutes more, transfer to bowls and serve.

Nutrition Facts Per Serving: Calories: 260; Fat: 12; Carbs: 17; Fiber: 13; Sugar: 5; Protein: 18

Paleo Eggplant Jam

(Prep + Cook Time: 1 hour 10 minutes | Servings: 6)

Ingredients:

- 3 eggplants; sliced lengthwise
- 2 tsp. sweet paprika
- 2 garlic cloves; minced
- A pinch of sea salt
- A pinch of cinnamon; ground
- 1tsp. cumin; ground
- A splash of hot sauce
- 1/4 cup water
- 1 tbsp. parsley; chopped
- 2 tbsp. lemon juice

Instructions:

1. Sprinkle some salt on eggplant slices and leave them aside for 10 minutes.
2. Pat dry eggplant slices, brush them with half of the oil, place on a lined baking sheet, place in the oven at 375 degrees F, bake for 25 minutes flipping them halfway and leave them aside to cool down.
3. In a bowl; mix paprika with garlic, cinnamon, cumin, water and hot sauce and stir well.
4. Add baked eggplant pieces and mash them with a fork.

5. Heat up a pan with the rest of the oil over medium-low heat, add eggplant mix, stir and cook for 20 minutes. Add lemon juice and parsley, stir; take off heat, divide into small bowls and serve.

Nutrition Facts Per Serving: Calories: 150; Fat: 3; Fiber: 2; Carbs: 6; Protein: 15

Stuffed Mushrooms

(Prep + Cook Time: 20 minutes | Servings: 4)

Ingredients:

- 12 big mushrooms; stems removed
- A pinch of sea salt
- Black pepper to the taste
- 1 small tomato; diced
- 1/4 cup homemade paleo pesto
- 2 tbsp. extra virgin olive oil

Instructions:

1. Brush mushrooms with the olive oil and season them with a pinch of sea salt and pepper to the taste.

2. Heat up a pan over medium high heat, add mushrooms and cook them for 5 minutes on each side. Transfer them to a platter, fill each with pesto sauce, top with diced tomatoes and serve.

Nutrition Facts Per Serving: Calories: 80; Fat: 4; Carbs: 5; Fiber: 0; Protein: 4

Celery Casserole

(Prep + Cook Time: 30 minutes | Servings: 8)

Ingredients:

- 1 white onion; finely chopped
- 1 celery head; chopped
- 2½ tbsp. ghee
- 1½ tbsp. coconut flour
- 1/2 tsp. nutmeg
- A pinch of sea salt
- Black pepper to the taste
- 1½ cups coconut milk
- 2 tbsp. extra virgin olive oil
- 1/2 cup flax meal

Instructions:

1. Heat up a pan with 1 tbsp. olive oil over medium high heat, add celery, stir and cook for a few minutes until it browns a bit.
2. Add a pinch of sea salt and pepper, stir and transfer to a baking dish.
3. Heat up the same pan with the rest of the olive oil over medium heat, add onions, stir and cook for 4 minutes.
4. Add 1½ tbsp. ghee, stir well and cook for 1-2 minutes.
5. Add coconut flour, stir well for a few minutes and take off heat.
6. Add coconut milk, pepper to the taste and nutmeg and stir very well.
7. Return to medium heat and stir for 2 minutes more.
8. Add the rest of the ghee and flax meal, stir and pour everything over celery.

9. Toss to coat, introduce in the oven at 350 °F and bake for 15

   minutes until it becomes golden. Take casserole out of the

oven, leave aside to cool down, cut, divide between plates

and serve.

Nutrition Facts Per Serving: Calories: 147; Fat: 9.2; Carbs: 11.3; Fiber: 1.5; Sugar: 2.1; Protein: 3.1

Paleo Potato Bites

(Prep + Cook Time: 40 minutes | Servings: 4)

Ingredients:

- 2 sweet potatoes; thinly sliced
- 1 cup salsa
- 4 oz. bacon; already cooked and crumbled
- 1 tsp. chili powder
- 1/2 tsp. garlic powder
- 1/2 tsp. paprika
- 2 tbsp. extra virgin olive oil
- Black pepper to the taste
- Some cilantro; finely chopped

For the guacamole:

- 1 tbsp. lime juice
- 2 avocados; pitted, peeled and chopped
- 1 garlic clove; minced
- 1/4 cup red onions; chopped
- 1/2 cup tomatoes; finely chopped

Instructions:

1. In a bowl; mix avocados with lime juice, garlic, red onions and tomatoes, stir well, cover and keep in the fridge for now.
2. In a bowl; mix potato slices with the olive oil, chili powder, garlic powder, paprika and pepper and toss to coat.
3. Spread potatoes on a lined baking sheet, introduce in the oven at 450 °F and bake for 10 minutes on each side.

4. Take potato slices out of the oven, top each with guacamole, bacon, salsa and chopped cilantro. Divide between plates and serve.

Nutrition Facts Per Serving: Calories: 240; Fat: 6; Carbs: 10; Fiber: 3; Sugar: 0.4; Protein: 17

Surprise Dinner Dish

(Prep + Cook Time: 1 hour 45 minutes | Servings: 5)

Ingredients:

- 1 paleo coconut bread; cubed
- 2 tbsp. ghee; melted
- 1 lb. sausage; casings removed
- 3 celery stalks; chopped
- 1 fennel; chopped
- 4 garlic cloves; chopped
- 1 yellow onion; chopped
- 8 oz. mushrooms; chopped
- 1 pear; chopped
- 1 red bell pepper; chopped
- 1 tbsp. thyme; chopped
- 2 tbsp. parsley; chopped
- 1/2 cup white wine
- A pinch of sea salt
- Black pepper to the taste
- 1 tsp. oregano; dried
- 3 eggs; whisked
- 2 cups chicken stock

Instructions:

1. Spread paleo bread cubes on a lined baking sheet, introduce in the oven at 300 degrees f and bake for 20 minutes.
2. Toss bread cubes, introduce in the oven again, bake for 20 minutes more, take out of the oven and leave aside for now.
3. Heat up a pan over medium high heat, add sausage, break with a fork, brown for a few minutes, transfer to a bowl and leave aside for now as well.
4. Return pan to medium high heat, add 1 tbsp. ghee, melt and add garlic, fennel, onion and celery, stir and cook for 10 minutes.

5. Transfer veggies to the bowl along with the sausage and stir everything.
6. Return the pan to medium high heat again, melt the rest of the ghee and add red pepper, mushrooms and wine.
7. Stir, cook until wine evaporates, take off heat and add this to the bowl with the veggies and the sausage.
8. Add thyme, oregano, a pinch of sea salt, pepper, parsley, bread cubes and 1½ cups stock, stir everything and leave aside for 10 minutes.
9. Add the rest of the stock and stir everything again.
10. Pour the veggies mix in a greased baking dish, spread whisked eggs all over, introduce in the oven at 400 degrees F, cover with tin foil and bake for 30 minutes.
11. Remove foil and bake for 15 more minutes. Divide between plates and serve.

Nutrition Facts Per Serving: Calories: 220; Fat: 12; Carbs: 5; Fiber: 0.6; Protein: 17.5

Veggie Mix And Scallops

(Prep + Cook Time: 14 minutes | Servings: 4)

Ingredients:

- 1 cup cauliflower rice; already cooked
- 1 tbsp. ginger; grated
- 2 mangos; peeled and chopped
- 1 cucumber; sliced
- 2 tsp. lime juice
- 1/2 cup cilantro; chopped
- 2 tsp. olive oil
- 1½ lbs. sea scallops
- Black pepper to the taste

Instructions:

1. In a bowl; mix cucumber slices with mangos, ginger, lime juice, half of the oil, cilantro and black pepper to the taste and stir well.
2. Pat dry scallops and season them with some pepper.

3. Heat up a pan with the rest of the oil over medium high heat, add scallops and cook for 2 minutes on each side. Divide scallops on plates, add cauliflower rice and mango and cucumber salad on the side and serve.

Nutrition Facts Per Serving: Calories: 180; Fat: 3; Fiber: 2; Carbs: 4; Protein: 14

Tomato And Mushroom Skewers

(Prep + Cook Time: 20 minutes | Servings: 4)

Ingredients:

- 1 lb. mushroom caps
- 4 cups cherry tomatoes
- 1 tbsp. raw honey
- Black pepper to the taste
- 2 tbsp. Dijon mustard
- 4 tbsp. extra virgin olive oil
- 4 garlic cloves; minced
- 1/2 cup cilantro; minced
- 1/4 cup ghee
- 1/2 cup parsley; minced

Instructions:

1. In a bowl; mix mustard with olive oil, pepper and honey and whisk well.
2. Arrange mushrooms and tomatoes on skewers alternating pieces, brush them with the mustard mix, arrange on preheated grill over medium high heat and cook for 3 minutes on each side.
3. Heat up apan with the ghee over medium high heat, add garlic, stir and cook for 3 minutes.

4. Add cilantro, parsley, salt and pepper to the taste and cook

   for 2 minutes more. Divide skewers on plates, drizzle herb

   sauce on top and serve.

Nutrition Facts Per Serving: Calories: 138; Fat: 5; Carbs: 15; Fiber: 0; Protein: 4

Broccoli And Cauliflower Fritters

(Prep + Cook Time: 20 minutes | Servings: 8)

Ingredients:

- 1 cup broccoli; chopped
- 1½ cups cauliflower; chopped
- A pinch of sea salt
- Black pepper to the taste
- 1 tbsp. coconut flour
- 2 eggs
- 1 tbsp. coconut oil for frying
- 2 tbsp. homemade mayonnaise
- 1 tbsp. extra virgin olive oil
- 1 tbsp. coriander; finely chopped
- 1/2 garlic clove; grated
- 1 tsp. lime juice

Instructions:

1. In a bowl; mix cauliflower with broccoli, eggs, coconut flour, a pinch of sea salt and pepper to the taste and stir very well.
2. Shape small patties and arrange them on a plate.
3. Heat up a pan with the coconut oil over medium high heat, add veggies fritters, cook for 4 minutes on each side, transfer them to paper towels, drain grease and arrange on a platter.

4. In a bowl; mix mayo with olive oil, coriander, garlic and lime

juice and stir well. Serve you fritters with mayo mix.

Nutrition Facts Per Serving: Calories: 140; Fat: 3.8; Carbs: 13; Fiber: 3.3; Sugar: 8; Protein: 7.3

Paleo Stuffed Zucchinis

(Prep + Cook Time: 30 minutes | Servings: 4)

Ingredients:

- 2 tomatoes; chopped
- 1 eggplant; chopped
- 2 zucchinis; cut into halves lengthwise
- 1 yellow onion; chopped
- A pinch of sea salt
- Black pepper to the taste
- 1/2 bunch parsley; finely chopped
- 3 tbsp. extra virgin olive oil
- 2 garlic cloves; minced

Instructions:

1. Remove flesh from zucchini halves, season them with a pinch of sea salt and pepper, leave aside for 10 minutes and pat dry them,
2. Heat up a pan with 1 tbsp. oil over medium high heat, add onion, stir and cook for 4 minutes.
3. Add garlic, stir and cook 1 minute. Add the rest of the oil, eggplant and chopped zucchini flesh, stir and cook for 10 minutes.
4. Add tomatoes, parsley and pepper to the taste, stir and cook for 5 minutes more.

5. Fill zucchini halves with this mix, place on preheated grill over medium high heat, cook for 3 minutes, divide between plates and serve right away.

Nutrition Facts Per Serving: Calories: 130; Fat: 6; Carbs: 9; Fiber: 2; Sugar: 0; Protein: 8

Stuffed Eggplant

(Prep + Cook Time: 1 hour 10 minutes | Servings: 2)

Ingredients:

- 1 eggplant
- 2 tomatoes; finely chopped
- 3 thyme springs
- 1 garlic clove; minced
- 3 tbsp. extra virgin olive oil
- A pinch of sea salt
- Black pepper to the taste
- Lemon juice from 1/2 lemon

Instructions:

1. Place eggplant on a lined baking sheet, introduce in the oven at 400 °F and bake for 30 minutes.
2. Take eggplant out of the oven, leave aside to cool down, cut in half lengthways, drizzle each half with 1 tbsp. olive oil, introduce in the oven again at 350 °F and bake for 25 more minutes.
3. Take eggplant halves out of the oven, leave aside for 5 minutes, discard flesh and sprinkle halves with some of the lemon juice, a pinch of sea salt and pepper.
4. In a bowl; mix tomatoes with thyme, garlic and chopped eggplant flesh and stir.

5. Add lemon juice, pepper and 1 tbsp. olive oil and stir everything well. Scoop this into eggplant halves, divide on a plate and serve.

Nutrition Facts Per Serving: Calories: 180; Fat: 22; Carbs: 8.5; Fiber: 3.4; Sugar: 2; Protein: 10

Cucumber Salsa

(Prep + Cook Time: 1 hour 10 minutes | Servings: 12)

Ingredients:

- 2 cucumbers; chopped
- 1/2 cup green bell pepper; chopped
- 2 tomatoes; chopped
- 1 jalapeno pepper; chopped
- 1 yellow onion; chopped
- 1 garlic clove; minced
- 2 tsp. cilantro; chopped
- 1 tsp. parsley; chopped
- 2 tbsp. lime juice
- 1/2 tsp. dill weed
- A pinch of sea salt
- Black pepper to the taste

Instructions:

1. In a bowl; mix cucumbers with jalapeno, tomatoes, green pepper, garlic, onion, a pinch of sea salt and pepper to the taste.

2. Add parsley, cilantro, dill and lime juice and stir well again.

   Keep in the fridge for 1 hour and serve.

Nutrition Facts Per Serving: Calories: 70; Fat: 0.2; Carbs: 1; Fiber: 2. protein 17

Delightful Falafel

(Prep + Cook Time: 65 minutes | Servings: 4)

Ingredients:

- 2 cups cauliflower florets
- 1 cup yellow onion; chopped
- 1 zucchini; chopped
- 1/2 cup parsley; chopped
- 4 garlic cloves; minced
- 1/4 tsp. chili powder
- 1/2 cup cilantro; chopped
- 2 tsp. cumin
- A pinch of sea salt
- Black pepper to the taste
- 1/2 cup almond flour
- 1/2 tsp. turmeric
- Zest from 1 lemon
- 1 egg; whisked
- Coconut oil

Instructions:

1. In your food processor, mix cilantro, onion, parsley and garlic, blend well and transfer to a bowl.
2. In your food processor, also mix cauliflower with zucchini, blend very well and pour over onion mix.
3. Add chili powder, lemon zest, cumin, turmeric, egg, almond flour, a pinch of salt and pepper to the taste and stir well.

4. Spread some coconut oil on a lined baking sheet, arrange falafels, introduce in the oven at 375 °F and bake for 40 minutes, brushing them with some more coconut oil halfway.

Nutrition Facts Per Serving: Calories: 230; Fat: 14; Carbs: 15; Fiber: 2; Protein: 22

Kohlrabi Dish

(Prep + Cook Time: 1 hour 10 minutes | Servings: 2)

Ingredients:

- 3 kohlrabi; peeled and thinly sliced
- A pinch of sea salt
- Black pepper to the taste
- 4 tbsp. ghee
- 1/3 cup parsley; chopped
- 2 tbsp. lard; melted

Instructions:

1. Arrange kohlrabi slices on the bottom of a baking dish.
2. Drizzle some of the lard over them, season with a pinch of salt and pepper and some of the parsley.
3. Add another layer of kohlrabi, drizzle more lard, season with pepper and parsley again and continue with kohlrabi slices again.
4. Finish with parsley.
5. Cover dish with tin foil, introduce in the oven at 350 °F and bake for 30 minutes.

6. Uncover dish, add ghee, introduce in the oven again and

   bake for 30 more minutes. Take the dish out of the oven,

   leave aside to cool down, slice, divide between plates and

   serve.

Nutrition Facts Per Serving: Calories: 207; Fat: 11; Carbs: 18; Fiber: 9.8; Sugar: 7; Protein: 11.1

Paleo Watercress Soup

(Prep + Cook Time: 30 minutes | Servings: 4)

Ingredients:

- 8 oz. watercress
- 1 tbsp. lemon juice
- A pinch of nutmeg; ground
- 4 oz. canned coconut milk
- A pinch of sea salt
- Black pepper to the taste
- 14 oz. veggie stock
- 1 celery stick; chopped
- 1 onion; chopped
- 1 tbsp. olive oil
- 12 oz. sweet potatoes; peeled and chopped

Instructions:

1. Heat up a pot with the oil over medium heat, add onion and celery, stir and cook for 5 minutes.
2. Add sweet potato pieces and stock, stir; bring to a simmer, cover and cook on a low heat for 10 minutes.
3. Add watercress, stir; cover pot again and cook for 5 minutes.

4. Blend this with an immersion blender, add a pinch of nutmeg, lemon juice, salt, pepper and coconut milk, bring to a simmer again, divide into bowls and serve.

Nutrition Facts Per Serving: Calories: 159; Fat: 8; Fiber: 3; Carbs: 6; Protein: 16

Paleo Stuffed Peppers

(Prep + Cook Time: 50 minutes | Servings: 4)

Ingredients:

- 1/4 cup ghee; melted
- 6 colored bell peppers
- 1 garlic head; cloves peeled and chopped
- 10 anchovy fillets
- 15 walnuts

Instructions:

1. Place bell peppers on a lined baking sheet, place in preheated broiler, cook for 20 minutes and leave them to cool down.
2. Heat up a pan with the ghee over low heat, add garlic, stir and cook for 10 minutes.
3. Grind walnuts in a coffee grinder and add this powder to the pan.
4. Also add anchovy and stir well.

5. Peel burnt skin off peppers, discard tops, cut in halves and

   remove skins. Divide pepper halves on plates, divide anchovy

   mix on them and serve.

Nutrition Facts Per Serving: Calories: 140; Fat: 3; Fiber: 3; Carbs: 6; Protein: 14

Baked Yuka With Tomato Sauce

(Prep + Cook Time: 35 minutes | Servings: 3)

Ingredients:

- 1 yucca root; cut into strips
- 1/2 tsp. garlic powder
- 2 tbsp. coconut oil
- Black pepper to the taste
- 1/2 tsp. smoked paprika
- 1/2 tsp. onion powder

For the sauce:

- 1 tomato; grated and skin discarded
- 1 garlic clove; grated
- 1 tbsp. vinegar
- 2 tbsp. extra virgin olive oil
- A pinch of sea salt

Instructions:

1. Put yucca strips in a bowl; drizzle with coconut oil, sprinkle pepper, garlic powder, onion powder and paprika, toss to coat, spread on a lined baking sheet, introduce in the oven at 390 °F and bake for 25 minutes.
2. Meanwhile; in a bowl, mix tomato with olive oil, a pinch of sea salt, vinegar and garlic and stir very well.

3. Take yucca out of the oven, transfer to plates and serve with

   tomato sauce drizzled on top.

Nutrition Facts Per Serving: Calories: 230; Fat: 2.7; Carbs: 51; Fiber: 2.5; Protein: 2

Onion Rings

(Prep + Cook Time: 21 minutes | Servings: 40 pieces)

Ingredients:

- 2/3 cup cashew meal
- A pinch of sea salt
- Black pepper to the taste
- 1 big red onion; sliced and rings separated
- 1 tsp. garlic powder
- 1/2 tsp. sweet paprika
- 1 tsp. onion powder
- 3 eggs

Instructions:

1. In a bowl; mix eggs with a pinch of sea salt and pepper and whisk well.
2. In another bowl; mix cashew meal with pepper, garlic and onion powder and sweet paprika and stir well.
3. Dip each onion ring in eggs and then in cashew meal mix, spread them on a lined baking sheet, introduce in the oven at 425 °F and bake for 10 minutes.

4. Transfer onion rings to preheated broiler and broil for 1 minute. Leave onion rings to cool down, divide between bowls and serve as a snack.

Nutrition Facts Per Serving: Calories: 134; Fat: 3.6; Carbs: 14; Fiber: 1.5; Protein: 4.5

Zucchini Noodles And Capers Sauce

(Prep + Cook Time: 10 minutes | Servings: 4)

Ingredients:

- 1 tbsp. capers; drained
- 1 garlic clove
- A pinch of sea salt
- Black pepper to the taste
- A pinch of red pepper flakes
- 15 kalamata olives; pitted
- 2 tbsp. olive oil
- 8 oz. cherry tomatoes; halved
- A handful basil; torn
- Juice of 1/2 lemon
- 4 zucchinis; cut with a spiralizer

Instructions:

1. In your food processor, mix capers with a pinch of sea salt, black pepper, pepper flakes and olives and blend well.

2. Transfer this to a bowl; add basil, oil and tomatoes, stir well and leave aside for 10 minutes. Divide zucchini noodles on plates, add tomatoes and capers sauce, toss to coat well and serve.

Nutrition Facts Per Serving: Calories: 100; Fat: 1; Fiber: 2; Carbs: 2; Protein: 6

Rutabaga Noodles And Cherry Tomatoes

(Prep + Cook Time: 35 minutes | Servings: 4)

Ingredients:

For the sauce:

- 1 tbsp. shallot; chopped
- 1 garlic clove; minced
- 3/4 cup cashews; soaked for a couple of hours and drained
- 2 tbsp. Nutritional yeast
- 1/2 cup veggie stock
- A pinch of sea salt
- Black pepper to the taste
- 2 tsp. lemon juice

For the pasta:

- 1 cup cherry tomatoes; halved
- 5 tsp. olive oil
- 1/4 tsp. garlic powder
- 2 rutabagas, peeled and cut into thin noodles

Instructions:

1. Place tomatoes and rutabaga noodles on a lined baking sheet, drizzle the oil over them, season with a pinch of sea salt, black pepper and garlic powder, toss to coat, place in the oven at 400 °F and bake for 20 minutes.
2. Meanwhile; in a food processor, mix garlic with shallots, cashews, veggie stock, Nutritional yeast, lemon juice, a pinch of sea salt and black pepper to the taste and blend well.

3. Divide rutabaga pasta between plates, top with tomatoes

   and drizzle the sauce over them.

Nutrition Facts Per Serving: Calories: 230; Fat: 2; Fiber: 5; Carbs: 10; Protein: 8

Paleo Eggplant Dish

(Prep + Cook Time: 50 minutes | Servings: 3)

Ingredients:

- 5 medium eggplants; sliced into rounds
- 1 tsp. thyme; chopped
- 2 tbsp. balsamic vinegar
- 1 tsp. mustard
- 2 garlic cloves; minced
- 1/2 cup olive oil
- Black pepper to the taste
- A pinch of sea salt
- 1 tsp. maple syrup

Instructions:

1. In a bowl; mix vinegar with thyme, mustard, garlic, oil, salt, pepper and maple syrup and whisk very well.

2. Arrange eggplant round on a lined baking sheet, place in the oven at 425 °F and roast for 40 minutes. Divide eggplants between plates and serve.

Nutrition Facts Per Serving: Calories: 120; Fat: 2; Fiber: 2; Carbs: 5; Protein: 15

Paleo Pancakes

(Prep + Cook Time: 25 minutes | Servings: 4)

Ingredients:

- 1/2 cup almond flour
- 1/2 cup tapioca flour
- Coconut oil for frying
- A pinch of sea salt
- Black pepper to the taste
- 1 cup coconut milk
- 1/2 tsp. chili powder
- 1/4 tsp. turmeric
- 1 small red onion; chopped
- 1 Serrano chili pepper; minced
- 1 small piece of ginger; grated
- A handful cilantro; chopped

Instructions:

1. In a bowl; mix almond and tapioca flour with milk, chili powder, a pinch of sea salt, pepper and turmeric and stir well.
2. Add onion, Serrano pepper, cilantro and ginger and stir very well.

3. Heat up a pan with the oil over medium high heat, pour 1/4 cup pancakes mix, spread, cook for 4 minutes on each side and transfer to a plate. Repeat with the rest of the batter and serve pancakes with green chutney.

Nutrition Facts Per Serving: Calories: 198; Fat 6.2; Carbs: 30; Fiber: 5.9; Sugar: 4; Protein: 8.5

Roasted Tomatoes

(Prep + Cook Time: 1 hour 10 minutes | Servings: 4)

Ingredients:

- 1 big red onion; cut into wedges
- 2 red bell peppers; chopped
- 2 garlic cloves; minced
- 1 lb. cherry tomatoes; halved
- 1 tsp. thyme; dried
- 1 tsp. oregano; dried
- 3 bay leaves
- 2 tbsp. olive oil
- 1 tbsp. balsamic vinegar
- A pinch of sea salt
- Black pepper to the taste

Instructions:

1. In a baking dish mix tomatoes with onions, garlic, a pinch of sea salt, black pepper, thyme, oregano, bay leaves, half of the oil and half of the vinegar, toss to coat, place in the oven at 350 °F and roast them for 1 hour.
2. Meanwhile; in your food processor, mix bell peppers with a pinch of sea salt, black pepper, the rest of the oil and the rest of the vinegar and blend very well.

3. Discard bay leaves, divide roasted tomatoes, garlic and onions on plates, drizzle the bell peppers sauce over them and serve.

Nutrition Facts Per Serving: Calories: 123; Fat: 1; Fiber: 1; Carbs: 2; Protein: 10

Sweet Potatoes And Cabbage Bake

(Prep + Cook Time: 1 hour 20 minutes | Servings: 4)

Ingredients:

- 8 sweet potatoes; cut into thin matchsticks
- 1 carrot; sliced
- 2½ cups green cabbage; shredded
- 2 garlic cloves; minced
- A pinch of sea salt
- Black pepper to the taste
- 4 oz. pancetta; chopped
- 3 tomatoes; sliced
- 1 tsp. thyme; dried

Instructions:

1. In a baking dish, mix cabbage with potatoes, garlic and carrot.
2. Add thyme, a pinch of sea salt and pepper and pancetta and toss to coat.
3. Spread tomato slices over veggie mix, cover dish with tin foil, introduce in the oven at 350 °F and bake for 35 minutes.

4. Discard tin foil and bake veggies for 30 more minutes. Take

   the dish out of the oven, leave aside to cool down, divide

   between plates and serve.

Nutrition Facts Per Serving: Calories: 190; Fat: 0.5; Carbs: 43; Fiber: 7; Protein: 5.9

Bell Peppers Stuffed With Tuna

(Prep + Cook Time: 20 minutes | Servings: 4)

Ingredients:

- 2 bell peppers; tops cut off, cut in halves and seeds removed
- 1 tbsp. capers; chopped
- 2 tbsp. tomato puree
- 4 oz. canned tuna; drained and flaked
- 1 scallion; chopped
- 1 tomato; chopped
- Black pepper to the taste

Instructions:

1. Place bell pepper halves on a lined baking sheet, place in preheated broiler over medium high heat, boil for 4 minutes and then leave them aside to cool down.
2. Meanwhile; in a bowl mix capers with tomato puree, tuna, tomato, black pepper and scallion and stir well.

3. Stuff bell peppers with this mix, place in preheated broiler again and cook for 5 minutes. Divide between plates and serve.

Nutrition Facts Per Serving: Calories: 140; Fat: 2; Fiber: 4; Carbs: 6; Protein: 15

Mexican Stuffed Peppers

(Prep + Cook Time: 30 minutes | Servings: 4)

Ingredients:

- 4 bell peppers; tops cut off and seeds removed
- 1/2 cup tomato juice
- 2 tbsp. jarred jalapenos; chopped
- 4 chicken breasts
- 1 cup tomatoes; chopped
- 1/4 cup yellow onion; chopped
- 1/4 cup green peppers; chopped
- 2 cups Paleo salsa
- A pinch of sea salt
- 2 tsp. onion powder
- 1/2 tsp. red pepper; crushed
- 1 tsp. chili powder
- 1/2 tsp. garlic powder
- 1/4 tsp. oregano
- 1 tsp. cumin; ground

Instructions:

1. In your slow cooker, mix chicken breasts with tomato juice, jalapenos, tomatoes, onion, green peppers, a pinch of salt, onion powder, red pepper, chili powder, garlic powder, oregano and cumin, stir well, cover and cook on Low for 6 hours.
2. Shred meat using 2 forks and stir everything well.

3. Stuff bell peppers with this mix, place them into a baking dish, pour salsa over them, place in the oven at 350 °F and bake for 20 minutes. Divide stuffed peppers on plates and serve.

Nutrition Facts Per Serving: Calories: 240; Fat: 4; Fiber: 3; Carbs: 7; Protein: 20

Grilled Cherry Tomatoes

(Prep + Cook Time: 36 minutes | Servings: 4)

Ingredients:

- 1 romaine lettuce head; chopped
- A handful basil; chopped
- 1 cucumber; sliced
- 3 handfuls spinach; chopped
- 2 avocados; pitted, peeled and cubed
- 2 scallions; chopped
- 1/2 cup almonds; chopped
- 3 handfuls green beans; blanched and chopped

For the tomatoes skewers:

- 3 tbsp. balsamic vinegar
- 24 cherry tomatoes
- 2 tbsp. olive oil
- 3 garlic cloves; minced
- 1 tbsp. thyme; chopped
- A pinch of sea salt
- Black pepper to the taste

For the salad dressing:

- 2 tbsp. balsamic vinegar
- A pinch of sea salt
- Black pepper to the taste
- 4 tbsp. olive oil

Instructions:

1. In a salad bowl; mix lettuce with spinach, cucumber, basil, avocado pieces, scallions, almonds and green beans.
2. In a smaller bowl; mix 4 tbsp. oil with 2 tbsp. balsamic vinegar, a pinch of sea salt and black pepper and whisk well.

3. Add this to salad, toss to coat and leave aside for now.
4. In a bowl; mix 2 tbsp. oil with 3 tbsp. vinegar, 3 garlic cloves, thyme, a pinch of sea salt and black pepper and whisk well.
5. Add tomatoes, toss to coat and leave aside for 30 minutes.
6. Drain marinade, skewer 6 tomatoes on one skewer and repeat with the rest of the tomatoes.

7. Place skewers on preheated grill over medium high heat, grill for 3 minutes on each side and divide between plates. Serve with the salad you've made earlier on the side.

Nutrition Facts Per Serving: Calories: 140; Fat: 1; Fiber: 1; Carbs: 2; Protein: 12

Paleo Avocado Spread

(Prep + Cook Time: 10 minutes | Servings: 4)

Ingredients:

- 2 avocados; pitted and peeled
- 4 bacon strips; cooked and crumbled
- 2 garlic cloves; minced
- 5 cherry tomatoes; halved
- 1 jalapeno pepper; chopped
- 1/2 red onion; chopped
- Juice of 1/2 lime
- A pinch of sea salt
- Black pepper to the taste

Instructions:

1. Put avocados in a bowl and mash them well.

2. Add garlic, jalapeno, onion, a pinch of salt, black pepper, lime juice and bacon and stir well. Top with cherry tomatoes halves and serve.

Nutrition Facts Per Serving: Calories: 140; Fat: 2; Fiber: 2; Carbs: 4; Protein: 12

Endive Bites

(Prep + Cook Time: 25 minutes | Servings: 4)

Ingredients:

- 4 slices bacon
- 16 endives leaves
- 2 tsp. white wine vinegar
- 1 cup cherry tomatoes; sliced
- A pinch of sea salt
- 1 tbsp. chives; chopped
- Black pepper to the taste
- 1 tbsp. extra virgin olive oil

Instructions:

1. Arrange bacon slices on a lined baking sheet, introduce in the oven at 400 °F and bake for 20 minutes.
2. Drain grease, transfer bacon to a cutting board, leave aside to cool down, crumble and put in a bowl.

3. In another bowl; mix tomatoes with chives, oil, a pinch of salt, pepper and vinegar and stir well. Divide this mix into endive leaves, sprinkle crumbled bacon on top of each, divide between plates and serve.

Nutrition Facts Per Serving: Calories: 120; Fat: 1; Carbs: 10; Fiber: 10; Sugar: 1; Protein: 6

Zucchini Noodles With Tomatoes And Spinach

(Prep + Cook Time: 30 minutes | Servings: 6)

Ingredients:

- 2 tbsp. olive oil
- 3 zucchinis; cut with a spiralizer
- 16 oz. mushrooms; sliced
- 1/4 cup sun dried tomatoes; chopped
- 1 tsp. garlic; minced
- 1/2 cup cherry tomatoes; halved
- 2 cups marinara sauce
- 2 cups spinach; chopped
- A pinch of sea salt
- Black pepper to the taste
- A pinch of cayenne pepper
- A handful basil; chopped

Instructions:

1. Put zucchini noodles in a bowl; season them with a pinch of salt and black pepper and leave them aside for 10 minutes.
2. Heat up a pan with the oil over medium high heat, add garlic, stir and cook for 1 minute.
3. Add mushrooms, stir and cook for 4 minutes.
4. Add sun dried tomatoes, stir and cook for 4 minutes more.
5. Add cherry tomatoes, spinach, cayenne, marinara and zucchini noodles, stir and cook for 6 minutes more. Sprinkle basil on top, toss gently, divide between plates and serve.

Nutrition Facts Per Serving: Calories: 120; Fat: 1; Fiber: 1; Carbs: 2; Protein: 9

Daikon Rolls

(Prep + Cook Time: 15 minutes | Servings: 4)

Ingredients:

- 1/2 cup pumpkin seeds
- 2 green onions; chopped
- 1/2 bunch cilantro; roughly chopped
- 2 tbsp. avocado oil
- 1 tbsp. lime juice
- 2 tsp. water
- A pinch of sea salt
- Black pepper to the taste
- 2 daikon radishes; sliced lengthwise into long strips
- 1 small cucumber; cut into matchsticks
- 1/2 avocado; pitted, peeled and sliced
- Handful microgreens

Instructions:

1. In your food processor, mix pumpkin seeds with a pinch of sea salt, pepper, cilantro and green onions and blend very well.
2. Add avocado oil gradually and lime juice and blend very well again. Add water and blend some more.

3. Spread this on each daikon slice, add cucumber matchsticks, avocado slices and micro greens, roll them, seal edges, divide between plates and serve.

Nutrition Facts Per Serving: Calories: 140; Fat: 0; Carbs: 23; Fiber: 0; Protein: 0

Cauliflower Pizza

(Prep + Cook Time: 40 minutes | Servings: 6)

Ingredients:

- 1½ cups mashed cauliflower
- A pinch of sea salt
- Black pepper to the taste
- 1/2 cup almond meal
- 1½ tbsp. flax seed; ground
- 2/3 cup water
- 1/2 tsp. oregano; dried
- 1/2 tsp. garlic powder
- Pizza sauce for serving
- Spinach leaves; chopped and already cooked for serving
- Mushrooms; sliced and cooked for serving

Instructions:

1. In a bowl; mix flax seed with water and stir well.
2. In a bowl; mix cauliflower with almond meal, flax seed mix, a pinch of sea salt, pepper, oregano and garlic powder, stir well, shape small pizza crusts, spread them on a lined baking sheet and bake them in the oven at 420 °F and bake for 15 minutes.

3. Take pizzas out of the oven, spread pizza sauce, spinach and mushrooms on them, introduce in the oven again and bake 10 more minutes. Divide between plates and serve.

Nutrition Facts Per Serving: Calories: 150; Fat: 8; Carbs: 20; Fiber: 1; Protein: 9

Paleo Tomato Quiche

(Prep + Cook Time: 30 minutes | Servings: 2)

Ingredients:

- 1 bunch basil; chopped
- 4 eggs
- 1 garlic clove; minced
- A pinch of sea salt
- Black pepper to the taste
- 1/2 cup cherry tomatoes; halved
- 1/4 cup almond cheese

Instructions:

1. In a bowl; mix eggs with a pinch of sea salt, black pepper, almond cheese and basil and whisk well.

2. Pour this into a baking dish, arrange tomatoes on top, place in the oven at 350 °F and bake for 20 minutes. Leave quiche to cool down, slice and serve.

Nutrition Facts Per Serving: Calories: 140; Fat: 1; Fiber: 1; Carbs: 2; Protein: 10

Spinach And Mushroom Dish

(Prep + Cook Time: 25 minutes | Servings: 2)

Ingredients:

- 6 mushrooms; chopped
- A handful cherry tomatoes; cut in halves
- 3 handfuls spinach; torn
- 1 tsp. ghee
- 2 tbsp. extra virgin olive oil
- 1 small red onion; sliced
- 1/2 tsp. lemon rind; diced
- 1 garlic clove; minced
- A pinch of sea salt
- Black pepper to the taste
- A pinch of nutmeg
- A drizzle of lemon juice

Instructions:

1. Heat up a pan with the ghee over medium high heat, add mushrooms, stir; cook for 4 minutes and transfer them to a plate.
2. Heat up the same pan with the olive oil over medium high heat, add onion, stir and cook for 3 minutes.
3. Add tomatoes, a pinch of sea salt, pepper, lemon rind, nutmeg and garlic, stir and cook for 3 minutes more.

4. Add spinach, stir and cook for 2-3 minutes. Add lemon juice at the end, stir gently, transfer to plates and serve with mushrooms on top.

Nutrition Facts Per Serving: Calories: 120; Fat: 4.5; Carbs: 7; Fiber: 2.5; Protein: 3.4

Paleo Liver Stuffed Peppers

(Prep + Cook Time: 25 minutes | Servings: 4)

Ingredients:

- 4 bacon slices; chopped
- 1 white onion; chopped
- 1/2 lb. chicken livers; chopped
- 4 garlic cloves; chopped
- 4 bell peppers; tops cut off and seeds removed
- A pinch of sea salt
- Black pepper to the taste
- 1/2 tsp. lemon zest; grated
- 1/4 tsp. thyme; chopped
- 1/4 tsp. dill; chopped
- A drizzle of olive oil
- A handful parsley; chopped

Instructions:

1. Heat up a pan over medium heat, add bacon, stir and cook for 2 minutes.
2. Add onion and garlic, stir and cook for 2 minutes.
3. Add livers, a pinch of salt and black pepper, stir; cook for 5 minutes and take off heat.
4. Transfer this to your food processor, blend very well, transfer to a bowl and aside for 10 minutes.

5. Add thyme, oil, parsley, lemon zest and dill, stir well and

   Stuff each bell pepper with this mix. Serve right away.

Nutrition Facts Per Serving: Calories: 150; Fat: 3; Fiber: 2; Carbs: 5; Protein: 12

Garlic Tomatoes

(Prep + Cook Time: 60 minutes | Servings: 4)

Ingredients:

- 4 garlic cloves; crushed
- 1 lb. mixed cherry tomatoes
- 3 thyme springs; chopped
- A pinch of sea salt
- Black pepper to the taste
- 1/4 cup olive oil

Instructions:

1. In a baking dish, mix tomatoes with a pinch of sea salt, black

   pepper, olive oil and thyme, toss to coat, place in the oven at

   325 °F and bake for 50 minutes. Divide tomatoes and pan

   juices between plates and serve.

Nutrition Facts Per Serving: Calories: 100; Fat: 0; Fiber: 1; Carbs: 1; Protein: 6

Paleo Cucumber Wraps

(Prep + Cook Time: 40 minutes | Servings: 4)

Ingredients:

For the mayo:

- 1 tbsp. coconut aminos
- 3 tbsp. lemon juice
- 1 cup macadamia nuts
- 1 tbsp. agave
- 1 tsp. caraway seeds
- 1/3 cup dill; chopped
- A pinch of sea salt
- Some water

For the filling:

- 1 cup alfalfa sprouts
- 1 red bell pepper; cut into thin strips
- 2 carrots; cut into thin matchsticks
- 1 cucumber; cut into thin matchsticks
- 1 cup pea shoots
- 4 Paleo coconut wrappers

Instructions:

1. Put macadamia nuts in a bowl; add water to cover, leave aside for 30 minutes and drain well.
2. In your food processor, mix nuts with coconut aminos, lemon juice, agave, caraway seeds, a pinch of salt and dill and blend very well.
3. Add some water and blend again until you obtain a smooth mayo.
4. Divide alfalfa sprouts, bell pepper, carrot, cucumber and pea shoots on each coconut wrappers, spread dill mayo over them, wrap, cut each in half and serve.

Nutrition Facts Per Serving: Calories: 140; Fat: 3; Fiber: 3; Carbs: 5; Protein: 12

Spaghetti Squash And Tomatoes

(Prep + Cook Time: 60 minutes | Servings: 4)

Ingredients:

- 1/4 cup pine nuts
- 2 cups basil; chopped
- 1 spaghetti squash; halved lengthwise and seedless
- Black pepper to the taste
- A pinch of sea salt
- 1 tsp. garlic; minced
- 1½ tbsp. olive oil
- 1 cup mixed cherry tomatoes; halved
- 1/2 cup olive oil
- 2 garlic cloves; minced

Instructions:

1. Place spaghetti squash halves on a lined baking sheet, place in the oven at 375 °F and bake for 40 minutes.
2. Leave squash to cool down and make your spaghetti out of the flesh.
3. In your food processor, mix pine nuts with a pinch of salt, basil and 2 garlic cloves and blend well.
4. Add 1/2 cup olive oil, blend again well and transfer to a bowl.

5. Heat up a pan with 1½ tbsp. oil over medium high heat, add tomatoes, a pinch of salt, some black pepper and 1 tsp. garlic, stir and cook for 2 minutes. Divide spaghetti squash on plates, add tomatoes and the basil pesto on top.

Nutrition Facts Per Serving: Calories: 150; Fat: 1; Fiber: 2; Carbs: 4; Protein: 12

Stuffed Baby Peppers

(Prep + Cook Time: 10 minutes | Servings: 4)

Ingredients:

- 12 baby bell peppers; cut into halves lengthwise and seeds removed
- 1/4 tsp. red pepper flakes; crushed
- 1 lb. shrimp; cooked, peeled and deveined
- 6 tbsp. jarred Paleo pesto
- A pinch of sea salt
- Black pepper to the taste
- 1 tbsp. lemon juice
- 1 tbsp. olive oil
- A handful parsley; chopped

Instructions:

1. In a bowl; mix shrimp with pepper flakes, Paleo pesto, a pinch of salt, black pepper, lemon juice, oil and parsley and whisk very well.

2. Divide this into bell pepper halves, arrange on plates and

   serve.

Nutrition Facts Per Serving: Calories: 130; Fat: 2; Fiber: 1; Carbs: 3; Protein: 15

Paleo Baked Eggplant

(Prep + Cook Time: 40 minutes | Servings: 3)

Ingredients:

- 2 eggplants; sliced
- A pinch of sea salt
- Black pepper to the taste
- 1 cup almonds; ground
- 1 tsp. garlic; minced
- 2 tsp. olive oil

Instructions:

1. Grease a baking dish with some of the oil and arrange eggplant slices on it.
2. Season them with a pinch of salt and some black pepper and leave them aside for 10 minutes.
3. In your food processor, mix almonds with the rest of the oil, garlic, a pinch of salt and black pepper and blend well.

4. Spread this over eggplant slices, place in the oven at 425 °F and bake for 30 minutes. Divide between plates and serve.

Nutrition Facts Per Serving: Calories: 140; Fat: 1; Fiber: 1; Carbs: 3; Protein: 15

Artichokes And Tomatoes Dip

(Prep + Cook Time: 40 minutes | Servings: 4)

Ingredients:

- 2 artichokes; cut in halves and trimmed
- Juice from 3 lemons
- 4 sun-dried tomatoes; chopped
- A bunch of parsley; chopped
- A bunch of basil; chopped
- 1 garlic clove; minced
- 4 tbsp. olive oil
- Black pepper to the taste

Instructions:

1. In a bowl; mix artichokes with lemon juice from 1 lemon, some black pepper and toss to coat.
2. Transfer to a pot, add water to cover, bring to a boil over medium high heat, cook for 30 minutes and drain.
3. In your food processor, mix the rest of the lemon juice with tomatoes, parsley, basil, garlic, black pepper and olive oil and blend really well.

4. Divide artichokes between plates and top each with the tomatoes dip.

Nutrition Facts Per Serving: Calories: 140; Fat: 1; Fiber: 1; Carbs: 3; Protein: 9

Paleo Cherry Mix

(Prep + Cook Time: 34 minutes | Servings: 4)

Ingredients:

- 1 tsp. coconut sugar
- 3 cups cherry tomatoes; halved
- 1/4 tsp. cumin; ground
- 1 tbsp. sherry vinegar
- A pinch of sea salt
- 1 red onion; chopped
- 2 cucumbers; sliced
- 1/4 cup olive oil
- Black pepper to the taste

Instructions:

1. Put cherry tomatoes in a bowl; season with coconut sugar, a pinch of salt and black pepper and leave aside for 30 minutes.
2. Drain tomatoes and pour juices into a pan.
3. Heat this up over medium heat, add cumin and vinegar and bring to a simmer.

4. Cook for 4 minutes, take off heat and mix with olive oil. Add

   tomatoes, onion and cucumber to this mix, toss well, divide

   between plates and serve.

Nutrition Facts Per Serving: Calories: 120; Fat: 1; Fiber: 2; Carbs: 2; Protein: 7

Stuffed Portobello Mushrooms

(Prep + Cook Time: 30 minutes | Servings: 4)

Ingredients:

- 10 basil leaves
- 1 cup baby spinach
- 3 garlic cloves; chopped
- 1 cup almonds; roughly chopped
- 1 tbsp. parsley
- 2 tbsp. Nutritional yeast
- 1/4 cup olive oil
- 8 cherry tomatoes; halved
- A pinch of sea salt
- Black pepper to the taste
- 4 Portobello mushrooms; stem removed and chopped

Instructions:

1. In your food processor, mix basil with spinach, garlic, almonds, parsley, Nutritional yeast, oil, a pinch of salt, black pepper to the taste and mushroom stems and blend well.

2. Stuff each mushroom with this mix, place them on a lined baking sheet, place in the oven at 400 °F and bake for 20 minutes. Divide between plates and serve right away.

Nutrition Facts Per Serving: Calories: 145; Fat: 3; Fiber: 2; Carbs: 6; Protein: 17

Zucchini Noodles And Pesto

(Prep + Cook Time: 20 minutes | Servings: 4)

Ingredients:

- 6 zucchinis; trimmed and cut with a spiralizer
- 1 cup basil
- 1 avocado; pitted and peeled
- A pinch of sea salt
- Black pepper to the taste
- 3 garlic cloves; chopped
- 1/4 cup olive oil
- 2 tbsp. olive oil
- 1 lb. shrimp; peeled and deveined
- 1/4 cup pistachios
- 2 tbsp. lemon juice
- 2 tsp. old bay seasoning

Instructions:

1. In a bowl; mix zucchini noodles with a pinch of sea salt and some black pepper, leave aside for 10 minutes and squeeze well.
2. In your food processor, mix pistachios with black pepper, basil, avocado, lemon juice and a pinch of salt and blend well.
3. Add 1/4 cup oil, blend again and leave aside for now.
4. Heat up a pan with 1 tbsp. oil over medium high heat, add garlic, stir and cook for 1 minute.
5. Add shrimp and old bay seasoning, stir; cook for 4 minutes and transfer to a bowl.
6. Heat up the same pan with the rest of the oil over medium high heat, add zucchini noodles, stir and cook for 3 minutes.
7. Divide on plates, add pesto on top and toss to coat well. top with shrimp and serve.

Nutrition Facts Per Serving: Calories: 140; Fat: 1; Fiber: 1; Carbs: 5; Protein: 14

Cucumber Noodles And Shrimp

(Prep + Cook Time: 25 minutes | Servings: 4)

Ingredients:

- 1 tbsp. Paleo tamari sauce
- 3 tbsp. coconut aminos
- 1 tbsp. sriracha
- 1 tbsp. balsamic vinegar
- 1/2 cup warm water
- 1 tbsp. honey
- 3 tbsp. lemongrass; chopped
- 1 tbsp. ginger; dried
- 1 lb. shrimp; peeled and deveined
- 1 tbsp. olive oil

For the cucumber noodles:

- 2 cucumbers; cut with a spiralizer
- 1 carrot; cut into thin matchsticks
- 1/4 cup balsamic vinegar
- 1/4 cup ghee; melted
- 1/4 cup peanuts; roasted
- 2 tbsp. sriracha sauce
- 1 tbsp. coconut aminos
- 1 tbsp. ginger; grated
- A handful mint; chopped

Instructions:

1. In a bowl; mix 3 tbsp. coconut aminos with 1 tbsp. vinegar, 1 tbsp. tamari, 1 tbsp. sriracha, warm water, honey, lemongrass, 1 tbsp. ginger, 1 tbsp. olive oil and whisk well.
2. Add shrimp, toss to coat and leave aside for 20 minutes.
3. Heat up your grill over medium high heat, add shrimp, cook them for 3 minutes on each side and transfer to a bowl.

4. In a bowl; mix cucumber noodles with carrot, ghee, 1/4 cup

   vinegar, 2 tbsp. Sriracha, 1 tbsp. coconut aminos, 1 tbsp.

   ginger, peanuts and mint and stir well. Divide cucumber

   noodles on plates, top with shrimp and serve.

Nutrition Facts Per Serving: Calories: 140; Fat: 1; Fiber: 2; Carbs: 3; Protein: 8

Stuffed With Beef

(Prep + Cook Time: 1 hour 5 minutes | Servings: 2)

Ingredients:

- 1 lb. beef; ground
- 1 tsp. coriander; ground
- 1 onion; chopped
- 3 garlic cloves; minced
- 2 tbsp. coconut oil
- 1 tbsp. ginger; grated
- 1/2 tsp. cumin
- 1/2 tsp. turmeric
- 1 tbsp. hot curry powder
- A pinch of sea salt
- 1 egg
- 4 bell peppers; cut in halves and seeds removed
- 1/3 cup raisins
- 1/3 cup walnuts; chopped

Instructions:

1. Heat up a pan with the oil over medium high heat, add onion, stir and cook for 4 minutes.
2. Add garlic, stir and cook for 1 minute.
3. Add beef, stir and cook for 10 minutes.
4. Add coriander, ginger, cumin, curry powder, a pinch of salt and turmeric and stir well.
5. Add walnuts and raisins, stir take off heat and mix with egg.

6. Divide this mix into pepper halves, place them on a lined baking sheet, place in the oven at 350 °F and bake for 40 minutes. Divide between plates and serve.

Nutrition Facts Per Serving: Calories: 240; Fat: 4; Fiber: 3; Carbs: 7; Protein: 12

Pork Stuffed Bell Peppers

(Prep + Cook Time: 36 minutes | Servings: 4)

Ingredients:

- 1 tsp. Cajun spice
- 1 lb. pork; ground
- 1 tbsp. olive oil
- 1 tbsp. tomato paste
- 6 garlic cloves; minced
- 1 yellow onion; chopped
- 4 big bell peppers; tops cut off and seeds removed
- A pinch of sea salt
- Black pepper to the taste

Instructions:

1. Heat up a pan with the oil over medium high heat, add garlic and onion, stir and cook for 4 minutes.
2. Add meat, stir and cook for 10 minutes more.
3. Add a pinch of salt, black pepper, tomato paste and Cajun seasoning, stir and cook for 3 minutes more.

4. Stuff bell peppers with this mix, place them on preheated grill over medium high heat, grill for 3 minutes on each side, divide between plates and serve.

Nutrition Facts Per Serving: Calories: 140; Fat: 3; Fiber: 2; Carbs: 3; Protein: 10

Carrots And Lime

(Prep + Cook Time: 40 minutes | Servings: 6)

Ingredients:

- 1¼ lbs. baby carrots
- 3 tbsp. ghee; melted
- 8 garlic cloves; minced
- A pinch of sea salt
- Black pepper to the taste
- Zest of 2 limes; grated
- 1/2 tsp. chili powder

Instructions:

1. In a bowl; mix baby carrots with ghee, garlic, a pinch of salt, black pepper to the taste and chili powder and stir well.
2. Spread carrots on a lined baking sheet, place in the oven at 400 °F and roast for 15 minutes.

3. Take carrots out of the oven, shake baking sheet, place in the oven again and roast for 15 minutes more. Divide between plates and serve with lime on top.

Nutrition Facts Per Serving: Calories: 100; Fat: 1; Fiber: 1; Carbs: 1; Protein: 7

Artichokes Dish

(Prep + Cook Time: 60 minutes | Servings: 4)

Ingredients:

- 16 mushrooms; sliced
- 1/3 cup tamari sauce
- 1/3 cup olive oil
- 4 tbsp. balsamic vinegar
- 4 garlic cloves; minced
- 1 tbsp. lemon juice
- 1 tsp. oregano; dried
- 1 tsp. rosemary; dried
- 1/2 tbsp. thyme; dried
- A pinch of sea salt
- Black pepper to the taste
- 1 sweet onion; chopped
- 1 jar artichoke hearts
- 4 cups spinach
- 1 tbsp. coconut oil
- 1 tsp. garlic; minced
- 1 cauliflower head; florets separated
- 1/2 cup veggie stock
- 1 tsp. garlic powder
- A pinch of nutmeg; ground

Instructions:

1. In a bowl; mix vinegar with tamari sauce, lemon juice, 4 garlic cloves, olive oil, oregano, rosemary, thyme, a pinch of salt, black pepper and mushrooms, toss to coat well and leave aside for 30 minutes.
2. Transfer these to a lined baking sheet and bake them in the oven at 350 °F for 30 minutes.
3. In your food processor, mix cauliflower with a pinch of sea salt and black pepper and pulse until you obtain your rice.

4. Heat up a pan over medium high heat, add cauliflower rice, toast for 2 minutes, add nutmeg, garlic powder, black pepper and stock, stir and cook until stock evaporated.

5. Heat up a pan with the coconut oil over medium heat, add onion, artichokes, 1 tsp. garlic and spinach, stir and cook for a few minutes. Divide cauliflower rice on plates, top with artichokes and mushrooms and serve.

Nutrition Facts Per Serving: Calories: 200; Fat: 3; Fiber: 2; Carbs: 7; Protein: 18

Warm Watercress Mix

(Prep + Cook Time: 20 minutes | Servings: 4)

Ingredients:

- 1 lb. watercress; chopped
- 1/4 cup olive oil
- 1 garlic clove; cut in halves
- 1 bacon slice; cooked and crumbled
- 1/4 cup hazelnuts; chopped
- Black pepper to the taste
- 1/4 cup pine nuts

Instructions:

1. Heat up a pan with the oil over medium heat, add garlic clove halves, cook for 2 minutes and discard.
2. Heat up the pan with the garlic oil again over medium heat, add hazelnuts and pine nuts, stir and cook for 6 minutes.

3. Add bacon, black pepper to the taste and watercress, stir; cook for 2 minutes, divide between plates and serve right away.

Nutrition Facts Per Serving: Calories: 100; Fat: 1; Fiber: 2; Carbs: 2; Protein: 6

Eggplant Hash

(Prep + Cook Time: 40 minutes | Servings: 4)

Ingredients:

- 1 eggplant; roughly chopped
- 1/2 cup olive oil
- 1/2 lb. cherry tomatoes; halved
- 1 tsp. Tabasco sauce
- 1/4 cup basil; chopped
- 1/4 cup mint; chopped
- A pinch of sea salt
- Black pepper to the taste

Instructions:

1. Put eggplant pieces in a bowl; add a pinch of salt, toss to coat, leave aside for 20 minutes and drain using paper towels.
2. Heat up a pan with half of the oil over medium high heat, add eggplant, cook for 3 minutes, flip, cook them for 3 minutes more and transfer to a bowl.
3. Heat up the same pan with the rest of the oil over medium high heat, add tomatoes and cook them for 8 minutes stirring from time to time.

4. Return eggplant pieces to the pan and also add a pinch of salt, black pepper, basil, mint and Tabasco sauce. Stir, cook for 2 minutes more, divide between plates and serve.

Nutrition Facts Per Serving: Calories: 120; Fat: 1; Fiber: 4; Carbs: 8; Protein: 15

Artichokes With Horseradish Sauce

(Prep + Cook Time: 55 minutes | Servings: 2)

Ingredients:

- 1 tbsp. horseradish; prepared
- 2 tbsp. mayonnaise
- A pinch of sea salt
- Black pepper to the taste
- 1 tsp. lemon juice
- 3 cups artichoke hearts
- 1 tbsp. lemon juice

Instructions:

1. In a bowl; mix horseradish with mayo, a pinch of sea salt, black pepper and 1 tsp. lemon juice, whisk well and leave aside for now.
2. Arrange artichoke hearts on a lined baking sheet, drizzle 2 tbsp. olive oil over them, 1 tbsp. lemon juice and sprinkle a pinch of salt and some black pepper.

3. Toss to coat well, place in the oven at 425 °F and roast them

   for 45 minutes. Divide artichoke hearts between plates and

   serve with the horseradish sauce on top.

Nutrition Facts Per Serving: Calories: 300; Fat: 3; Fiber: 12; Carbs: 16; Protein: 10

Paleo Stuffed Poblanos

(Prep + Cook Time: 50 minutes | Servings: 4)

Ingredients:

- 2 tsp. garlic; minced
- 1 white onion; chopped
- 10 poblano peppers; one side of them sliced and reserved
- 1 tbsp. olive oil
- Cooking spray
- 8 oz. mushrooms; chopped
- A pinch of sea salt
- Black pepper to the taste
- 1/2 cup cilantro; chopped

Instructions:

1. Place poblano boats in a baking dish which you've sprayed with some cooking spray.
2. Heat up a pan with the oil over medium high heat, add chopped poblano pieces, onion and mushrooms, stir and cook for 5 minutes.
3. Add garlic, cilantro, salt and black pepper, stir and cook for 2 minutes.

4. Divide this into poblano boats, introduce them in the oven at

   375 °F and bake for 30 minutes. Divide between plates and

   serve.

Nutrition Facts Per Serving: Calories: 150; Fat: 3; Fiber: 2; Carbs: 4; Protein: 10

Paleo Purple Carrots

(Prep + Cook Time: 1 hour 10 minutes | Servings: 2)

Ingredients:

- 6 purple carrots; peeled
- A drizzle of olive oil
- 2 tbsp. sesame seeds paste
- 6 tbsp. water
- 3 tbsp. lemon juice
- 1 garlic clove; minced
- A pinch of sea salt
- Black pepper to the taste
- White and sesame seeds

Instructions:

1. Arrange purple carrots on a lined baking sheet, sprinkle a pinch of salt, black pepper and a drizzle of oil, place in the oven at 350 °F and bake for 1 hour.
2. Meanwhile; in your food processor, mix sesame seeds paste with water, lemon juice, garlic, a pinch of sea salt and black pepper and pulse really well.

3. Spread this over carrots, toss gently, divide between plates

   and sprinkle sesame seeds on top.

Nutrition Facts Per Serving: Calories: 100; Fat: 1; Fiber: 1; Carbs: 5; Protein: 10

Garlic Sauce

(Prep + Cook Time: 20 minutes | Servings: 4)

Ingredients:

- 2 tbsp. avocado oil
- 2 garlic cloves; minced
- 3 eggplants; cut into halves and thinly sliced
- 1 red chili pepper; chopped
- 1 green onion stalk; chopped
- 1 tbsp. ginger; grated
- 1 tbsp. coconut aminos
- 1 tbsp. balsamic vinegar

Instructions:

1. Heat up a pan with half of the oil over medium high heat, add eggplant slices, cook for 2 minutes, flip, cook for 3 minutes more and transfer to a plate.
2. Heat up the pan with the rest of the oil over medium heat, add chili pepper, garlic, green onions and ginger, stir and cook for 1 minute.

3. Return eggplant slices to the pan, stir and cook for 1 minute.

   Add coconut aminos and vinegar, stir; divide between plates

   and serve.

Nutrition Facts Per Serving: Calories: 130; Fat: 2; Fiber: 4; Carbs: 7; Protein: 9

Paleo Carrot Hash

(Prep + Cook Time: 55 minutes | Servings: 4)

Ingredients:

- 1 tbsp. olive oil
- 6 bacon slices; chopped
- 3 cups carrots; chopped
- 3/4 lb. beef; ground
- 1 yellow onion; chopped
- A pinch of sea salt
- Black pepper to the taste
- 2 scallions; chopped

Instructions:

1. Place carrots on a lined baking sheet, drizzle the oil, season with a pinch of salt and some black pepper, toss to coat, place in the oven at 425 °F and bake for 25 minutes.
2. Meanwhile; heat up a pan over medium high heat, add bacon and fry for a couple of minutes.
3. Add onion and beef and some black pepper, stir and cook for 7-8 minutes more.

4. Take carrots out of the oven, add them to the beef and bacon mix, stir and cook for 10 minutes. Sprinkle scallions on top, divide between plates and serve.

Nutrition Facts Per Serving: Calories: 160; Fat: 2; Fiber: 1; Carbs: 2; Protein: 12

Eggplant Casserole

(Prep + Cook Time: 60 minutes | Servings: 4)

Ingredients:

- 2 eggplants; sliced
- 3 tbsp. olive oil
- 1 lb. beef; ground
- 1 garlic clove; minced
- 3/4 cup tomato sauce
- 1/2 bunch basil; chopped
- A pinch of sea salt
- Black pepper to the taste

Instructions:

1. Heat up a pan with 1 tbsp. oil over medium high heat, add eggplant slices, cook for 5 minutes on each side, transfer them to paper towels, drain grease and leave them aside.
2. Heat up another pan with the rest of the oil over medium high heat, add garlic, stir and cook for 1 minute.
3. Add beef, stir and cook for 5 minutes more.
4. Add tomato sauce, stir and cook for 5 minutes more.
5. Add a pinch of sea salt and black pepper, stir; take off heat and mix with basil.
6. Place one layer of eggplant slices into a baking dish, add one layer of beef mix and repeat with the rest of the eggplant slices and beef.

7. Place in the oven at 350 °F and bake for 30 minutes. Leave eggplant casserole to cool down, slice and serve.

Nutrition Facts Per Serving: Calories: 342; Fat: 23; Fiber: 7; Carbs: 10; Protein: 23

Grilled Artichokes

(Prep + Cook Time: 35 minutes | Servings: 4)

Ingredients:

- 2 artichokes; trimmed and halved
- Juice of 1 lemon
- 1 tbsp. lemon zest grated
- 1 rosemary spring; chopped
- 2 tbsp. olive oil
- A pinch of sea salt
- Black pepper to the taste

Instructions:

1. Put water in a pot, add a pinch of salt and lemon juice, bring to a boil over medium high heat, add artichokes, boil for 15 minutes, drain and leave them to cool down.
2. Drizzle olive oil over them, season with black pepper to the taste, sprinkle lemon zest and rosemary, stir well and place them on your preheated grill.

3. Grill artichokes over medium high heat for 5 minutes on each

   side, divide them between plates and serve.

Nutrition Facts Per Serving: Calories: 120; Fat: 1; Fiber: 2; Carbs: 6; Protein: 7

Incredible Glazed Carrots

(Prep + Cook Time: 25 minutes | Servings: 4)

Ingredients:

- 1 lb. carrots; sliced
- 1 tbsp. coconut oil
- 1 tbsp. ghee
- 1/2 cup pineapple juice
- 1 tsp. ginger; grated
- 1/2 tbsp. maple syrup
- 1/2 tsp. nutmeg
- 1 tbsp. parsley; chopped

Instructions:

1. Heat up a pan with the ghee and the oil over medium high heat, add ginger, stir and cook for 2 minutes.
2. Add carrots, stir and cook for 5 minutes.

3. Add pineapple juice, maple syrup and nutmeg, stir and cook

   for 5 minutes more. Add parsley, stir; cook for 3 minutes,

   divide between plates and serve.

Nutrition Facts Per Serving: Calories: 100; Fat: 0.5; Fiber: 1; Carbs: 3; Protein: 7

Paleo Breakfast

Tasty scramble

Serves 1

Ingredients

1 small clove garlic, minced

2 kale leaves, shredded

2 pastured eggs

2 tablespoons coconut oil

Radish and clover sprouts to top

2 radishes grated

1 pinch cayenne pepper

1 tablespoon turmeric

Directions

1. Heat a pan and lightly sauté garlic in coconut oil.

2. Crack eggs into the pan and cook until scrambled.

3. Once almost done, add in turmeric, shredded kales, and cayenne.

4. If desired, top with the sprouts and radish.

Frozen breakfast muffins

Serves 4

Ingredients

1 gallon freezer bag

2 cups banana

½ cup coconut milk, unsweetened

¼ cup coconut oil

1 cup sliced strawberries, frozen

2 teaspoons maple syrup

1 tablespoon flaxseed, ground

⅓ cups almond flour

½ cups dates

Directions

1. Line muffin tins and then add ground flax, almond meal and dates into a food processor.

2. Pulse the mixture to make it crumbly and transfer to a bowl. Then stir in maple syrup. Press a tablespoon of crust mixture into the button of the muffin gently, to create a crust.

3. Put semi-thawed strawberries into a food processor and pulse to smoothness. Add in coconut oil and coconut milk slowly until you achieve a thick, sorbet consistency.

4. Into a bowl, pour the strawberries and gently fold in the bananas. Then sub-divide the straw-berry banana over the top of bread crust evenly.

5. Put the muffin into a freezer and let it freeze and solidify. Once done, remove from the muffin tins and let it thaw for 10 additional minutes before you serve.

Breakfast Salad

Serves: 1-2

Ingredients

Oil for frying the eggs

2 eggs

¼ teaspoon sea salt

1 tablespoon olive oil

¼ cup of pine nuts, toasted

1 small handful of parsley, roughly chopped

1 small handful of fresh basil, chopped

1 not too ripe avocado, diced

1 red pepper, diced

147

2 large handfuls of cherry tomatoes, halved

½ English cucumber, thickly sliced

Directions

1. Into a large bowl, combine together olive oil, pine nuts, all veggies and salt and toss well.

2. Over medium heat, heat a cast iron or a skillet and add a splash of oil. Once the pan is hot, add eggs to the pan.

3. Once done remove the eggs from the skillet and serve with the salad.

Ham Stir-Fry

Serves 2

Ingredients

1 medium avocado, diced

¼ teaspoon black pepper, freshly ground

½ pound ham, diced

1/8 teaspoon thyme

1 small sweet potato, diced into ¼ inch cubes

4 medium mushrooms, sliced

¼ medium yellow onions, diced

1 tablespoon   coconut oil

Directions

1. Over medium heat, heat a large sauté pan and then add in coconut oil. Follow with thyme, sweet potatoes, mushrooms and onions.

2. Cook until the sweet potatoes are tender. Ensure you stir regularly.

3. Add in a few drops of water to the pan, cover and continue cooking.

4. Toss the ham until it's heated through, and then season using fresh ground pepper.

5. Now top with an avocado and serve.

Almond "Oatmeal"

Serves 2

Ingredients

1 teaspoon nutmeg, fresh, grated

1 teaspoon cinnamon, to taste

2 tablespoons canned coconut milk, full fat, unsweetened

4 tablespoons almond butter, raw, chunky

1 ½ cups applesauce, unsweetened

Directions

1. Into a pan over medium heat, add all the ingredients and heat until warm. Ensure that you stir often until well incorporated.

2. Now add in the dried or fresh fruits or the nuts to improve flavor.

Breakfast Burger

Serves 4

Ingredients

1lb ground turkey or beef

2 teaspoons basil

5 eggs

1 teaspoon minced garlic

8 slices cooked bacon

2 tablespoons almond meal

2 sun dried tomatoes cut into small pieces

½ cup ground sausage

Directions

1. Mix the beef or turkey with sun-dried tomatoes, 1 egg, garlic, almond meal, basil and form 4 burger patties.

2. Cook the burger patties in a skillet for around five minutes or each side or until done then transfer to plates.

3. Now fry the sausage in a skillet then top the burgers with sausage then bacon.

4. Fry the remaining four eggs then place on top of the burgers.

Paleo Lunch

Paleo Burrito

Serves: 3-4

Ingredients

2 teaspoon cumin, ground

2 teaspoons smoked paprika

1 ½ tablespoon chili powder

1 4.5 oz can diced green chilies

1 14.5 oz can diced tomatoes

1 lb ground beef, preferably grass fed

2 cloves garlic, minced

⅓ cup celery, chopped

⅓ cup bell pepper, chopped

⅓ cup onion, chopped

3 cups broccoli slaw

2 tablespoons olive oil

Salt and Pepper

Cilantro and avocado, for garnish

Directions

1. Sauté celery, bell pepper, onions, broccoli slaw and garlic in olive oil until you get preferred tender crispness. After around 6-8 minutes, set aside.

2. Then brown the ground beef; drain and add the spices, green chilies and tomatoes.

3. Put a layer of vegetables on a plate and top with the meat sauce. Sprinkle some cilantro, and try other toppings like salsa, green onions or jalapenos if desired.

Sardine Stuffed Avocado

Serves 1-2

Ingredients

¼ teaspoon Himalayan salt

1 teaspoon turmeric root, freshly ground

1 tablespoon fresh lemon juice

1 medium spring onion or bunch chives

1 tablespoon mayonnaise

1 tin sardines, drained

1 large avocado

Directions

1. Cut the avocado into half and remove its pit. Then drain the sardines and put them in a bowl.

2. Scoop the flesh from the avocado half but leave a ½-1 inch of avocado flesh. Then add in spring onions finely sliced and ground turmeric root. The follow with mayonnaise and combine well.

3. Now add in the scooped avocado flesh and, mash to your preferred smoothness, and squeeze in fresh lemon juice and salt.

4. To serve, scoop the avocado mixture into each avocado half.

Garlic Chicken And Cherry Tomato-Sauce
Serves: 4-6

Ingredients

¼ teaspoon pepper

½ teaspoon salt

1 ½ teaspoons crushed basil

1 ½ lbs cherry tomatoes

2 lbs chicken cutlets

1 tablespoon chopped garlic- about 4 cloves

¾ cup diced red onion

2 tablespoon olive oil

Directions

1. Over medium heat, heat oil in a large skillet and then add in onion and garlic. Cook for about 5 minutes and use a spatula to regularly mix the ingredients.

2. To the pan, add in the chicken and cook for about 3-4 minutes on each side to brown. Thicker chicken breasts may take longer; say 6-8 minutes.

3. Into a food processor, chop the cherry tomatoes and add to the pan with the chicken, and combine together.

4. Then add in pepper, salt and basil and bring to a boil. Allow to simmer for about 25 minutes before serving.

Raw Vegan Tacos

Serves 4-5

Ingredients

1 avocado, sliced

½ cup cilantro, chopped

½ zucchini, shredded

½ purple onion, diced

1 large tomato, seeded and diced

3 tablespoons olive oil

1 serrano pepper, sliced

1 garlic clove, minced

1/8 teaspoon cayenne pepper

½ teaspoon chili powder

2 teaspoons coriander

2 teaspoons cumin

2 cups raw walnuts

1 head iceberg lettuce

Nutritional yeast to taste

Salt and pepper to taste

Directions

1. Rinse the lettuce, drain and set aside. Into a food processor, place the walnuts and pulse to ground fully.

2. Add in Serrano pepper, garlic, cayenne pepper, chili powder, coriander, cumin and olive oil and continue to pulse to incorporate the mixture.

3. Cut the bottom of iceberg lettuce, and slice the head into two. To reveal the cups, pull apart the layers gently.

4. Into the cups, spoon walnut mixture and top with diced tomatoes, chopped cilantro, shredded zucchini and onion.

5. Slide in a few avocado slices, and season with salt and pepper. Top with nutritional yeast and serve.

Kale Salad

Serves 2-3

Ingredients for the salad

½ red onion, very thinly sliced

2 bunches kale, or 6 packed cups of baby kale

6 Medjool dates, pitted

1/3 cup whole hazelnuts

For the dressing

5 tablespoons toasted hazelnut oil

Pinch of coarse salt

1 medjool date

4 tablespoons orange juice, freshly squeezed

2 tablespoons apple cider vinegar

Directions

1. Preheat the oven to 375 degrees and then put hazelnuts into a baking dish. Roast for about 7-8 minutes, to have the skin darken and begin to split.

2. Transfer the nuts to a kitchen towel, wrap them, then steam for 15 minutes.

3. Immediately they cool, squeeze and twist around firmly to remove the skin, still wrapped in the towel.

4. Into a food processor, put the hazelnuts and pulse until finely chopped. Set aside to top the salad.

5. Wash, dry and chop the kales and then put in a large bowl. Slice the onion thinly and add into the bowl.

6. Prepare the dressing by combining the ingredients for dressing in a blender apart from the oil. Puree to break down the dates and then drizzle the oil in a steady stream to emulsify the dressing.

7. Toss the kale and onion mixture alongside the orange-hazel nut dressing. Transfer into a platter bowl and sprinkle with the hazelnut and dates mixture.

Kale And Meatball Soup

Serves 5-6

Ingredients

3 cups of spinach, roughly chopped

3 cups of kale, roughly chopped

6 cups water

1-28 oz can whole, stewed tomatoes

1 teaspoon paprika

½ tablespoon dried oregano

½ tablespoon coriander

½ tablespoon cumin

1 jalapeno, minced

3 cloves of garlic, minced

1 onion, chopped

1 tablespoon olive oil

Salt to taste

Meatball Ingredients

1 tablespoon olive oil

1 teaspoon black pepper

1 teaspoon cayenne pepper

1/2 tablespoon salt

1/2 tablespoon garlic powder

1 tablespoon oregano, dried

1 tablespoon fennel seeds

1 egg

1 lb. lean ground beef

Directions

1. Into a large bowl, combine the egg, spices and beef and shape into 2 inch meatballs.

2. Heat oil in a large frying pan and sear the meatballs on all sides, and turn them after 3 minutes.

3. As the meatballs cook, dice and mince jalapeno, garlic and onion to use for the base of soup. Season this with some salt.

Heat olive oil in a large pot and cook the base for 7 minutes over medium heat, until soft.

4. Add the paprika, oregano, coriander and cumin and stir, and then add tomatoes. Crush them up together with their juices from the can.

5. Let the base simmer and then pour the meatballs to the pot. Use a little water to deglaze the frying pan and add to the pot. Add 6 cups of water and bring to a boil.

6. Taste the soup and season with salt if desired, and then add spinach and kales. You can serve soon after the greens have cooked through.

Paleo Dinner

Chicken Puttanesca With Artichokes

Serves 4

Ingredients

2 tablespoon fresh parsley, chopped

¼ cup fresh basil, chopped

1 tablespoon capers, chopped

¼ cup kalamata olives, chopped

1 14.5-oz can salt-free artichoke hearts, halved

1 14.5-oz can tomatoes, no-salt-added

1 tablespoon anchovy paste

1 tablespoon red pepper, crushed

½ tablespoon thyme, dried

3 cloves garlic, minced

1 yellow bell pepper, diced

¼ cup white wine

1 large yellow onion, diced

Salt and pepper

2 8-oz boneless, skinless chicken breasts, halved

1 tablespoon olive oil, divided

Directions

1. Into a large pan, heat a tablespoon of oil over medium heat.

2. Use salt and pepper to season the chicken breast and cook for about 5-7 minutes. Once it browns, remove from heat and put onto a plate.

3. To the pan, add the remaining oil and then reduce the heat to medium. Add onions and sauté for around 2 minutes and follow with bell pepper. In case the brown onion bits appear to burn, deglaze with white wine.

4. Once the sautéed onions are transparent and soft, add in anchovy paste, red pepper, dried thyme and garlic. Cook the mixture for a minute as you stir, until it turns fragrant.

5. Now add in the capers, olives, tomatoes and the remaining wine; and then allow to simmer.

6. Put back the chicken to the pan; add in the sauce and chicken juices. Cover and simmer the mixture for about 20 minutes.

7. Once the sauce is slightly reduced the chicken is cooked through, stir in the fresh herbs; and adjust the seasoning based on your preferred taste.

Creamy Coconut Shrimp "Pasta"

Serves 2

Ingredients

2 large zucchinis, peel on, stringed

¼ teaspoon garam masala

Juice of 1 lime

¼ cup fresh cilantro, chopped

½ cup coconut cream

300g cooked shrimp

1 small onion, very finely chopped

225g mushrooms, sliced

½ teaspoon black pepper, freshly cracked

½ teaspoon fine sea salt or Himalayan

1 cup pure coconut water

¾ cup water

600g cauliflower, roughly chopped

Directions

1. Onto a medium saucepan, add in pure coconut water, water and cauliflower and bring to a boil. Reduce the heat and cook while covered for about 5-7 minutes to fully soften the cauliflower.

2. Into a large skillet, cook the mushrooms until golden, then add in pepper, salt and onions and continue to cook until soft and fragrant.

3. Into the blender, ladle the cauliflower mixture and process on high speed to achieve a smooth and silky consistency.

4. Now pour the cauliflower mixture over the onions and mushrooms and add in garam masala, lime juice, coconut cream and cooked shrimp.

5. Over low-medium heat, bring the mixture to a simmer to warm the shrimp and then stir in fresh cilantro.

6. To serve, divide the stringed zucchini into 2 plates and ladle shrimp sauce over it

Avocado, Arugula Salad With Pan Seared Fish

Serves: 2

Ingredients for *Salad*

1 tablespoon flax seeds

1 ruby red grapefruit or orange, chilled

1 large avocado

1 bunch arugula or baby arugula

For Dressing

¼ teaspoon black pepper

1 tablespoon miso

2 tablespoons honey

¼ tablespoon olive oil

½ cup apple cider vinegar

The Fish

1 egg

2 filets of tilapia (omit the flour if using Salmon)

¼teaspoon salt

1 tablespoon Cajun seasoning

½ cup almond flour

Directions

1. Onto a plate, put Cajun seasoning and almond flour and mix well.

2. Into a bowl, break the egg and beat; and then dredge the fish filet through the egg. Use the flour and Cajun seasoning mixture to cover both sides. Shake off the excess and then set aside.

3. Prepare a large bowl, and then wash and spin dry the arugula. Put it into the bowl.

4. Into a jar, place the dressing ingredients, seal and shake to combine. Pour ¼ cup of the arugula and flax seeds then toss to cover. Put the arugula onto a serving plate.

5. Cut the grape fruit into sections or wheels, and the avocado into slices. Place the slices alternately in a circle on top of the arugula, and add a little more dressing.

6. Heat 1-2 tablespoons of olive oil in a stainless steel pan on high heat. Wait until the oil is hot then add filet in the pan. Cook until it lifts easily from the pan.

7. Flip the filet over and cook for 2 additional minutes while uncovered.

8. Add ¼ cup of water into the pan then cook the fish. Once cooked, put the fish onto the salad and enjoy.

Chicken Breast With Citrus

Serves 4

Ingredients

1 10 ounce can cherry tomatoes

1 small onion, cut into wedges

2 small oranges that are sliced crosswise

1 large lime, cut into wedges

1 teaspoon ground pepper

2 large chicken breasts

For Sauce

¼ teaspoon salt

1 garlic clove, minced

1 teaspoon cumin, ground

2 tablespoons fresh parsley, finely chopped

3 tablespoons of finely chopped fresh oregano

3 tablespoons olive oil

¼ cup fresh lime juice

¼ cup fresh orange juice

Directions

1. Into a small bowl, whisk together the sauce ingredients.

2. Fry the chicken breast and then pound them down into even thickness of 1/3 inches.

3. Into a food storage bag or medium bowl, pour half of the Mojo sauce over the chicken as a marinade. Cover the bowl or seal the bag.

4. Cover the sauce that remains and put under refrigeration for at least two hours. Meanwhile heat the indoor grill pan to medium-high or the outdoor grill to around 400 F degrees.

5. Remove the chicken from the marinade, discard the marinade, and then season chicken with salt and pepper. Grill each side of the chicken for 4 minutes each until no-longer pink in the center.

6. Take out the chicken from the pan and add in the onions, oranges and limes and grill for 3 more minutes, as you stir occasionally. Add in the tomatoes, and grill for 1-2 minutes to soften.

7. To serve, drizzle with the stored sauce.

Chicken Pesto-Zucchini Pasta

Serves 4

Ingre-di-ents

4 oz Red Sauce (tomato sauce)

4 zuc-chini

4 Chicken Breasts

4 tablespoons Basil Pesto

Fresh Pep-per to taste

Himalayan Sea Salt

Directions

1. First season the chicken with salt and pepper and then grill over medium heat. Meanwhile have water simmering in a pot to steam the zucchini.

2. Then warm up the red sauce and maintain it at low simmer, and slice the zucchini length-wise to obtain thin strips.

3. Steam the zucchini just about 3 minutes before the chicken is cooked through.

4. Onto a plate spoon the red sauce, and toss zucchini with the pesto; then place onto the red sauce.

5. Slice the chicken and put it over the zucchini and then serve.

Red Sauce

Ingre-di-ents

Fresh pep-per to taste

Himalayan sea salt

1 oz coconut oil

1 teaspoon basil, dried

1 teaspoon thyme, dried

1 teaspoon oregano, dried

4 gar-lic cloves, minced

4 onions, minced

4 28oz cans of plum tomatoes

Directions

1. In a large pot, sauté onions in oil on low heat, until it turns translucent.

2. Add in garlic and herbs, and continue to cook for a few minutes then remove from heat.

3. Then add in tomatoes and use an immersion blender to puree.

4. Simmer the mixture until it's reduced to about 2/3rd, and then add in salt and pepper to taste.

5. Serve immediately or alternatively cool in the freezer.

Basil Pesto

Ingre-di-ents

Fresh Pep-per to taste

Himalayan Sea Salt

3 cloves garlic

¼ cup pine nuts

½ cup extra vir-gin olive oil

3 bunches basil

Directions

1. Into a food processor, add garlic and basil leaves. Mix together and add olive oil, followed by pine nuts.

2. Taste and season with salt and pepper as desired.

White Turkey Chili

Serves: 4-6

Ingredients

½ teaspoon onion powder

½ teaspoon garlic powder

2 teaspoons cumin

2 ½ teaspoons ancho chili powder

1 onion

1 poblano pepper

1 tablespoon olive oil

2 cups cooked turkey

4 cups of turkey broth

1 cup of water

1 head of cauliflower

Optional Garnish:

Chopped tomatoes

Avocado

Cilantro

Directions

1. Add a cup of water into a large stockpot and then set the heat to high.

2. Chop the cauliflower roughly and put it into the water stockpot. Once the water begins to boil; lower the heat to medium.

3. Cook while covered for 10-12 minutes to soften the cauliflower; as you occasionally check if more water will be needed. Meanwhile, add olive oil into a skillet and set the heat to medium.

4. Then coarsely chop the onions and add to the olive oil, to cook for around 3-5 minutes.

5. Prepare the poblano pepper by chopping and removing the seeds, and dice. Add it to the onions and then cook for 3-4 more minutes.

6. Now chop the already cooked turkey.

7. Then drain the cauliflower and add it with the broth into a blender, and process to smoothness.

8. Add in the turkey, onions, peppers and spices and cook for 5-10 minutes. Serve and enjoy.

Honey Salmon With Roasted Fennel

Serves 1

Ingredients

2 tablespoons shaved almonds

2 teaspoons pure local honey

2 8-oz wild salmon filets

Lemon juice

Sea salt

Olive oil

1 fennel bulb

Roasted Fennel

Directions

1. Preheat your oven to around 400 degrees F.

2. Cut the stems of the fennel, which you can preserve for garnish or soups if desired. Then chop the white bulb into chunks and drizzle with olive oil, pepper, and salt.

3. While uncovered, roast the fennel for around 30 minutes, and then spread the honey on salmon filets then top with shaved almonds.

4. Onto a roasting or baking pan, place the salmon with the skin side facing down. After the fennel has been in the oven for 30 minutes, pop the salmon.

5. Bake both until the fish is cooked through and almonds browned. This should take around 12 minutes.

Paleo Desert

Pumpkin Pie Smoothie

Serves 2

Ingredients

1/8 teaspoon cinnamon

1/8 teaspoon ginger

¼ teaspoon vanilla extract

1 teaspoon maple syrup

1/8 teaspoon allspice

1/8 teaspoon nutmeg

1 ½ cups almond milk, unsweetened

½ cup pumpkin puree

1 ½ frozen banana

Directions

1. Place all the ingredients apart from cinnamon, into a blender and blend on high until smooth.

2. Then transfer the smoothie into a glass and garnish with cinnamon. Serve and enjoy.

Avocado Mint 'Ice Cream'

Serves 2

Ingredients

1 tablespoon honey

½ cup full fat coconut milk

½ teaspoon peppermint extract

1 cup chopped, frozen banana

½ ripe green avocado

Directions

1. Puree all ingredients in a food processor, to create a thick and smooth paste.

2. Pour into a bowl and place in a freezer while covered, for around 2 hours, and ensure that you stir every 30 minutes.

3. Once you have achieved the desired consistency, remove from the freezer and serve.

Chocolate Buns

Serves: 8

Ingredients

¼ cup sultanas (golden raisins)

½ teaspoon bicarb soda

¼ cup cacao powder

½ cup coconut flour

¼ cup orange juice

¼ cup honey

½ cup coconut milk

4 eggs

Directions

1. First preheat the oven to 340 degrees F; and use coconut oil to grease 8 muffin tins.

2. Use an electric beater to beat the eggs for a minute, then add in honey, orange juice and coconut milk. Beat a second time.

3. Add in the cacao powder, bicarb soda and coconut flour and combine using an electric beater for one minute.

4. Stir through the sultanas and then scoop the batter into muffin tins.

Bake the buns for around 17-20 minutes.

Paleo Brownie

Serves 4

Ingredients

1 teaspoon coconut oil, softened

1-2 inches mashed banana

1 tablespoon almond milk, unsweetened

1 egg white

2 teaspoons cocoa powder

1 teaspoon chocolate chips

1 teaspoon coconut flour

3 tablespoons Almond Meal

Directions

1. Preheat the oven to 350 degrees Fahrenheit

2. Meanwhile, spray a ramekin or a small baking dish with non-stick cooking spray and set aside.

3. Smash a banana in a medium sized bowl, add egg white, almond milk, coconut oil and mix.

4. Combine the ingredients until the texture of the contents resembles the typical brownie batter.

5. Into a baking dish, transfer the batter and bake at 350 degrees Fahrenheit.

6. After about 22-25 minutes, check whether the middle is well cooked. Stick a toothpick and check whether it comes out dry, and then serve.

Chocolate Cake

Serves 8

Ingredients

Cake

1/3 cup coconut oil

½ cup coconut flour

1 teaspoon vanilla

1/3 cup + 1 tablespoons arrowroot flour

1 teaspoon distilled white vinegar

5 tablespoons unsweetened cocoa powder

½ cup almond milk

1 teaspoon cinnamon

½ cup water

1 teaspoon baking soda

1 cup honey

¾ teaspoon baking powder

1 cup honey

6 eggs

Frosting

½ teaspoon pure vanilla

1/3 cup unsweetened cocoa powder

1 10-ounce package dairy free chocolate chips

168

1/3 cup water

2 tablespoons honey

1 cup Earth balance butter

Directions

1. Preheat the oven to 350 degrees then line 2 (8-inch) pie pans with parchment paper and grease with coconut oil then dust with cocoa powder and put aside.

2. Mix together the milk and vinegar in a large bowl then put in the fridge.

3. In another bowl, whisk the coconut flour, cinnamon, salt, arrowroot flour, baking soda and baking powder then put aside.

4. Bring the water to a boil in a saucepan and once it starts to boil, remove it from the heat then add in cocoa powder and coconut oil then stir until smooth and nicely melted.

5. Remove the milk from the fridge then add in eggs, vanilla, and honey and stir.

6. Now stir the cocoa mixture into the dry ingredients then add the egg mixture and beat until there are no lumps.

7. Pour the butter into two pans then back for 30 minutes or until the cake center springs back on touch then allow to cool.

To make frosting:

1. Put the cocoa powder in a bowl then bring the water to boil. Pour the water over the cocoa powder then stir until smooth and set aside.

2. Put the chocolate chips in a microwavable bowl then hat for around 25 seconds, stir then repeat until the chocolate is melted and smooth.

3. Beat the butter and honey until fluffy for around five minutes then add the cooled cocoa mixture, vanilla, and melted chocolate then mix well.

4. Add the frosting once the cake cools down.

Paleo Snacks

Cucumber Noodles With Blueberries

Serves: 6-8

Ingredients

1 cup cilantro leaves

2 cups blueberries

¼ cup olive oil

¼ teaspoon cumin, ground

1 clove garlic, finely chopped

4 teaspoons lime juice, fresh

2 large jalapeño chilies, seeded and finely chopped

4 large cucumbers

Salt

Directions

1. Use a julienne peeler to prepare cucumber noodles.

2. Mix together olive oil, cumin, garlic, lime juice and jalapeno in a large bowl.

3. Then add in cilantro, blueberries and cucumber noodles and toss to coat.

Garlicky Zoodles With Slivered Almonds

Serves

Ingredients

¼ cup slivered almonds

Salt & pepper

Pinch red pepper flakes

3-4 tablespoons garlic olive oil

3 large zucchini, peeled and ends removed

Directions

1. Cut the ends of the zucchini, peel and spiralize using the vegetable slicer.

2. Into a large skillet, heat oil and add almond, pepper, salt and red pepper. Cool for 10 minutes as you stir until it turns tender.

3. Remove the mixture into a serving plate or tray and then sprinkle with almonds that remained. Serve.

Barbecue Zucchini Chips

Serves: 6-8

Ingredients

Olive oil

3 zucchini

½ teaspoon black pepper

½ teaspoon mustard

½ teaspoon cumin

1 teaspoon paprika

1 teaspoon garlic powder

1 tablespoon sea salt

1-2 tablespoons coconut sugar, to taste

1 tablespoon chili powder

Directions

1. Preheat your oven to 300 degrees F.

2. In a small bowl, combine cayenne, black pepper, mustard, cumin, paprika, garlic, sea salt, coconut sugar and chili powder to prepare a barbecue spice blend.

3. Slice the zucchini to create 1/8 inch slices, and mist the olive oil over the zucchini slices. Then sprinkle the spice blend over the slices of zucchini and bake for 4o minutes.

4. Take out from the oven, flip the slices and mist some olive oil on the other side. Then sprinkle the spice blend over the other side.

5. Bake for around 2o minutes, but take care not to over-bake.

Paleo Seed Bars

Serves 12

Ingredients

4 tablespoons sesame seeds

2 tablespoons chia seeds

100g sunflower seeds

100g pumpkin seeds

1 teaspoon cinnamon

Pinch of salt

4 tablespoons tahini

2 tablespoons coconut oil plus more for greasing

1 ripe banana

Directions

1. Blend the banana, tahini, coconut oil, cinnamon, and salt until you have a paste then add in the rest of the ingredients and pulse for another minute or so.

2. Pour this mixture into a cake tin greased with coconut oil then put in the freezer for an hour.

3. After the hour, remove it from the freezer, cut into bars then return it to the fridge. These tasty snacks can last week.

Tahini And Mustard Crackers

Makes 15 crackers

Ingredients

2 ½ tablespoons coconut flour

1 tablespoon wholegrain mustard

Pinch of salt

2 tablespoons sesame seeds

1 egg

1 tablespoon coconut oil

3 tablespoons tahini paste

Directions

1. Preheat oven to 338°F.

2. Mix egg, tahini, coconut oil, salt, mustard, sesame seeds in a bowl until well mixed. Now add in coconut flour mix until thick and sticky.

3. Roll mixture into a ball and put on a greased parchment paper then flatten it using your hands until it is flat then cover this with a piece of parchment paper then flatten it using a rolling pin into a thin dough layer.

4. Use a knife to make small incision marks horizontally and vertically in order for the crackers to cook.

5. Place this in the middle shelf to cook for around 15 minutes. Since the outer are likely to cook faster, I recommend that you remove the tray once they start browning then slice the edges off, return to oven and cook for another 5 minutes.

6. Let the crackers cool before breaking apart.

Conclusion

Thank you again for downloading this book!

I hope this book was able to help you to learn more about the paleo diet and get started with the amazing recipes.

The next step is to start by getting rid of all the foods you should not eat and stock your pantry with foods that you should eat so that preparing the food becomes easier.

Thank you and good luck!

Part 2

Introduction

This book was designed for the real beginner and the absolute beginner to the Paleo Diet. It talks about the diet from a very basic point of view. Don't expect a lot of technical details included.

The book also includes some practical steps to help you get started on the diet – or at least to try it for a few days. In fact, I have included tips, recipes, and even a simple meal plan that beginners and anyone curious can try for just 3 days.

That way you can get a feel if you can live the Paleo way or not.

Thank you again for downloading this book, I hope you like it!

Chapter 1: What Is The Paleo Diet?

Back in the year 2013 the term "Paleo Diet" was Google's number one search term when it comes to weight loss. Some people learned about it from the Internet while others became aware of such a diet through celebrity endorsements.

When you have names like Gwyneth Paltrow, Grant Hill, Matthew McConaughey, Megan Fox, and Jessica Biel among many others who are on the diet you just have to try it. Some of them are even strong and vocal promoters of the diet. Some have maintained their figures with the help of the diet.

So What is the Paleo Diet Anyway?

The Paleo diet, or more correctly – the Paleo way of eating – simply means mimicking the diet available to cavemen during the Paleolithic era (thus the name of the diet). Simply put – if a certain food item wasn't available to the folks during the Paleo era many thousands of years ago then you can't eat it.

This diet is also known by other names such as the caveman diet, Paleolithic diet, hunter-gatherer diet, evolutionary diet, ancestral diet, and primal diet, among others. All these names are descriptive of what this way of eating is like. It's primal because it's very simple and basic.

It's called the hunter-gatherer diet simply because you eat the food that can be hunted or gathered – yes you're not supposed to eat anything that is produced by modern agriculture (more of that in the next chapter). I learned about it simply because I wanted to find a way to lose weight.

Benefits of the Paleo Diet

Weight Loss: There are folks on the Paleo diet who are in it for weight loss. I found it surprising that the Paleo diet includes a lot of fat (including animal fat!), nuts, and other fat sources. However, as it was explained to me, it was all within the context.

I used to eat bacon and ham as a part of meals that are tasty yet increased my risk of heart disease.

In the Paleo diet, I still ate bacon but it was part of an anti-inflammatory strategy. I no longer ate it with highly processed food. I ate it with healthy fruits and veggies thus in the long run it helped me lose weight and maintain my figure.

Now there are those who say that science does not back the diet. Of course they will say that but did they ever mention actual medical studies on the Paleo Diet? There are studies like this and this one that affirm the weight loss effects of following this diet.

Note that anyone can go on any diet for a few days and lose weight. But that is just water weight not your actual weight – you can get your water weight back pretty soon. But if you check out the long term effects of the diet you'll find that the Paleo Diet actually helps you lose weight.

On top of that, it isn't a restrictive diet. I still eat a lot of the food that I like to eat. If you live on a protein heavy diet like me then you'll love the Paleo lifestyle.

Cardio Health, Lactose Intolerance, Improved Metabolism, and Diabetes: Some folks are on the Paleo diet because it helps them improve their cardiovascular health. The people that I know who have diabetes are on the diet because it is beneficial to their health. But don't get me wrong, there are studies like this one and this one that shows how beneficial this diet is to people who have these particular health issues.

It Contributes to Muscular Gain: some people live the Paleo lifestyle simply because they want to build more muscle. Note that this diet includes a lot of animal meat (check out the list of food that you can and cannot eat in the next chapter). The more muscle you gain the faster your metabolism.

Improved Gut Health: Another added benefit of this diet is better gut health. You're immediately kicking out all the junk food from your system. Any inflammation in your intestinal tract caused by processed food will eventually go away in time.

Chapter 2: Paleo Dos And Don'ts

If you're in it for weight loss just like me then may be the Paleo Diet is just right for you. I particularly don't like calorie counting, which is why I have failed in the other diets I have tried. The good news is that the Paleo diet doesn't make you do any calorie counts.

I never had to count how many calories I've had nor have I tried to figure out if I'm lacking in any nutrient. There are no nutrient counts in the Paleo Diet. I just eat when I'm hungry and stop eating when I'm full. There's no need to binge or sneak to the fridge at night just get a midnight snack.

It's not a highly restrictive diet! However, there are a few dos and don'ts that you have to follow. As stated in the first chapter, the rules of the Paleo way of eating (some people refuse to call it a diet, since it really isn't a "diet" in the popular sense of the word nowadays).

Paleo Dos

It's all very simple really. All you need to do is to eat healthy fats and oils (this came as an initial shock to me since I just finished with a zero fat diet), spices, herbs, seeds, nuts, fruits, vegetables, eggs, fish (lots of it), and a lot of meat. Note that that meat sources should be grass fed so you better check if the cow, that is now your steak was fed, was allowed to graze naturally or not.

Paleo Don'ts

The number one thing that the Paleo Diet condemns (I know, it's such a strong word) is processed food. Any type of processed food should be avoided – so check the label next time you go to the grocery. Anything that has a weird sounding name on the label or any ingredient that you find difficult to pronounce should not be inside your cart.

Other than processed foods you shouldn't have any trans fats in your diet – yes, it's the unhealthy fats that tend to clog your circulatory system. Margarine and all types of vegetable oils are also out. All types of artificial sweeteners are also prohibited – that means all cola drinks are out.

Legumes and dairy products also have to go (a big nod of approval for folks who are lactose intolerant). And another big shock to me is that grains are not allowed in this diet. Well, there weren't any grains during the Paleolithic era. They didn't have agriculture back then so there was no way for the cave man to mass produce wheat, barley, rice, and other grains.

That also means you're not supposed to get any store bought pasta and bread. However, there are Paleo approved ingredients that you can use to make bread. Some people ask where they will get their energy from – it should be common knowledge now that carbs from grains is the basic source of energy in our modern diet.

Well, the answer to that question is in the protein that you consume. That's where you get your calories. The healthy fat that you eat is also another source of energy – it's also a really good source of calories. You're actually just switching from one energy source for another albeit healthier source.

Now, I can put a really long food list in this book but that would defeat the purpose of teaching you to figure out if something is Paleo or not. Here's a little golden rule that you should remember when you're doing your groceries:

"If the food in front of you can't be hunted or gathered by our cavemen ancestors then don't eat it."

That means you should go to the aisles that have all the processed food. You'll be forced to walk to the outer rim of the grocery store where all the natural food is found.

Chapter 3: How To Get Started On The Paleo Diet

Now that you know the dos and don'ts and a host of other things about the Paleo diet, the next question is how you actually get started. We'll go over the different adjustments that you will have to make in this chapter. In the following chapter we'll outline a simple 5 day meal plan so you'll know what an actual Paleo week will be like.

From there you can make your own meal plans so you won't have to fuss about what food you have to prepare each day. And to help ensure that you don't eat anything that isn't Paleo, here is a step by step action plan on how to get started on the diet.

Step 1 – Get the Bags and Boxes Ready

Prepare a huge bag or box. This is where you will put all the food that you have in store that isn't Paleo. You don't have to throw the food away – that's big waste. If you have a neighbor that will be willing to take the food you will remove from your premises then give it to them. You can even donate the food to charity. There will be lots of soup kitchens that will be willing to take the food and other ingredients.

You can separate each type of food item in a separate container so they will be easier to identify – that is if you are donating them. Make sure to arrange everything properly inside the box since some of the items may spill if you're not careful. Of course, leftovers will go directly to the trash. Don't even think about get one last hurrah out of the left overs, that will be dishonest of you.

Step 2 – Time to Clear the Kitchen

Go over the stuff in your kitchen. Start with the most obvious place – the fridge! Open the fridge and say goodbye to all non-

Paleo items in there. Anything that has refined sugars, legumes, tubers, anything that's obviously starchy, all types of beans, any form of processed meat in the freezer should go. All types of processed food inside the fridge should go.

Next check your cupboards. Look for grains like rice, wheat, corn, and others. Pack them separately in different containers and then place them inside your box. Since grains usually are the heaviest food items they should go all the way to the bottom of the container. Look for oils that are taboo in the Paleo diet. This includes cottonseed oil, soybean oil, peanut oil, and corn oil among other things. If you still have peanut butter then you should seal that and pack it away.

Step 3 – Stock Up on Paleo Stuff

The next step is to deliver your box of non-Paleo goodies and give them away. It's up to you who you want to give it to. The important thing is that in switching to this new diet you are also able to bless or benefit someone who may be in need. Once you're done clearing your drawers, cupboards, cabinets, cellars, and the fridge it's time to go to do some groceries.

You'll need lots of protein sources – make sure they're the grass fed ones! You can get pork, duck, chicken, venison, beef and even wild game. Of course you'll need fish and other types of seafood as well. Don't forget to get some tuna, shrimp, salmon, tilapia, perch, cod, and others.

Don't forget to stock up on veggies, herbs, and fruits as well. That includes potatoes, tomatoes, bell peppers, garlic, some greens, mushrooms, and many more. Don't forget oranges, bananas, mangoes, cantaloupes, peaches, plums, blueberries and others. Nuts and seeds will also be a staple so add them to your grocery list. Other items that you shouldn't forget include coconut milk and coconut oil – make sure you have them in your list.

Step 4 – Live a Hunter Gatherer Lifestyle

Eating Paleo won't be that effective if you tend to eat everything that's in the fridge. Here's an idea – eat only when you're hungry. That's how our ancestors did it. They stocked up on food, yes, but they only ate when they're hungry.

In order to help you get over your hunger pangs (note: your body will crave and even want to get the good old dose of fructose and other processed sugars), you need to prepare a pretty stuffing meal. For instance, if 1 portion of meat isn't enough for you then make it two portions next time.

You can also add an extra portion of veggies and an extra portion of fruit just to make each meal a lot more filling. Oh yes, you can also get a double portion of fat. In case you're planning your meals and you decide to wing it and not follow a meal plan for that day just remember to include meat + veggies + fruit + fat into your next meal; you'll never go wrong with that.

What If You Can't Get Over Certain Paleo Items?

Some people find it difficult to let go of certain food items – like dairy, ice cream, cereal, or rice (a particular issue for some Asians that I know of). The good news is that you don't have to force yourself. While you're still in the transition from your old diet to this new one, you can skip one food group or food item at a time.

If you have a particular liking for sodas and colas for instance, you can start by reducing the amount of cola you're having each day until you can go without it on certain days. Make sure to find substitutes. For instance, if you love having bread in the morning so much, you can substitute Paleo approved flour sources like coconut flour and almond flour, arrow root powder, coconut flakes etc.

You can continue removing one non-Paleo item from your pantry at a time. You don't have to be absolutely strict about it at first. Try to condition your body until you no longer need to have it.

Chapter 4: Sample Paleo Recipes

Now that you have an idea about what the Paleo Diet is, what types of food are allowed (and what aren't), as well as the benefits of going Paleo, we'll list down a few recipes that might help you get a picture of what you will be eating in case you do decide to try it. You can try the recipes here and see if you can live off of the meals.

The good news about going Paleo is that it is a very sustainable eating plan – some people don't want to call it a diet, remember? The meals aren't really that restrictive. You'll have to quit a lot of highly processed food, of course, but in exchange you'll get really tasty full meals. Check out the recipes below if you're not convinced.

Now, honestly, some Paleo recipes may be a bit time consuming to prepare. However, there are other Paleo recipes that only take a minute to cook. You actually have a wide array of options when you make your meal plans. That's a big plus, actually.

Sample Breakfast Recipes

Breakfasts are always a rush for many folks. However, there are days, like weekends and holidays, when you can take your sweet time and prepare a feast. We have included a variety of Paleo breakfast recipes here – some you can prepare in just a few minutes.

Stuffed Peppers

If you love eating eggs then you'll love this recipe. It uses bell pepper cups and each one is stuffed with an egg and some spinach. It's the perfect power breakfast to start a demanding day.

Ingredients:

- Pepper
- Sea salt
- Eggs (medium size, 4 pieces)
- Spinach (16 ounces – chopped)
- *Bell peppers (4 pieces, regular or large size – any color)*

Instructions:

Preheat your oven up to 300 degrees Fahrenheit. Get some foil and use it to line a baking dish. To make the bell pepper cups, slice off the tops of each bell pepper, remove all the seeds inside. Grab the baking dish and place the peppers in it. Bake them for only 15 minutes.

While waiting, chop the spinach. After 15 minutes, remove the peppers from the oven. Fill the peppers halfway through with the chopped spinach. Crack an egg and fill each pepper with one egg. Add salt and pepper to taste.

Bake stuffed peppers for 15 minutes. Serve and enjoy.

English Muffins

If you can't have enough of eggs then get eggs with bacon (it's perfectly legal in the Paleo diet!). And what better way to complete the meal than to have some muffins along. Here's a quick English muffin recipe – Paleo style. This cooks under 5 minutes.

Ingredients:

- Water (2 tablespoons)
- Coconut oil (1 teaspoon)
- Egg (1 regular size)
- Kosher salt (1/8 teaspoon)
- Baking soda (1/4 teaspoon)
- Coconut flour (1 tablespoon)
- *Cashew flour (1/4 cup)*

Instructions:

Mix together all dry ingredients in one container. Whisk them until everything is well combined. Add all wet ingredients. Mix thoroughly until you get a nice and even texture. Grease a ramekin (make sure to use one that is microwave safe). Place mixture in ramekin. Microwave the mixture for 2 minutes.

Allow it to cool. Slice your fresh Paleo muffin into two equal halves. Toast each half for a couple of minutes – do that using a toaster oven. Serve with egg and bacon.

Eggs Benedict

If you're big on brunches then this recipe is one of the best Paleo options for your family. This recipe makes 4 servings.

Ingredients:

- Chives
- Pepper
- Salt
- Olive oil
- Garlic clove (1 piece)
- Red onion (1 regular size)
- Pre-cooked sausage links (4 pieces; lengthwise slices)
- **Eggs (4 poached; 4 egg yolks for sauce)**

Ingredients for Hollandaise Sauce:

- Egg yolks (4 pieces
- Lemon juice (1 tablespoon)
- Salt (1 teaspoon)
- Cayenne pepper (1/8 teaspoon)
- **Warmed ghee 1/2 cup)**

Instructions:

Preheat oven to 400 degrees Fahrenheit. Peel and chop potatoes into small pieces. Slice onions into wedges. Mince garlic. Split sausage links. Give sausages and veggies a toss in olive oil. Line baking sheet and spread ingredients evenly.

Season the mixture with pepper and salt to taste. Top with herbs.

Bake in oven for 30 minutes. Top with poached eggs then serve with Hollandaise sauce.

Instructions for Hollandaise Sauce:

Make the Hollandaise sauce by whisking cayenne, salt, lemon juice, and egg yolks. When the ingredients have combined into a thick mixture, blend them slowly in a food processor. Drizzle warmed ghee slowly as the ingredients get mixed well.

Paleo Pancakes

Enjoy pancakes in the morning – with a twist! You'll be using bananas as natural sweeteners. Here's how.

Ingredients:

- Bananas (2 pieces, regular sized)
- Eggs (4 pieces, regular size)
- Almond butter (2 teaspoons)
- *Chocoloate chips (see Paleo chocolate bits recipe)*

Instructions:

Mash bananas and then mix in almond butter. Add eggs. Mix well until you get an even consistency (I sometimes just put everything in a blender especially when I don't have that much time).

Heat a flat pan. Scoop up about ¼ cup of the mixture and cook it in the pan. Wait for bubbles to appear on top and then turn/flip the pancake. Each side will only take a minute to cook. Add some chocolate chips/bits on top. You can also add some fresh fruit on top before serving – if you wish.

Sample Paleo Lunch Recipes

Lunch recipes ala Paleo are just as filling as any other "regular" lunch recipe. Some recipes can be considered gourmet type ones while others can be considered as home cooked meals.

189

Check out the recipes I have included here – I have also included my favorites! They're all easy to make and some of them only have 200 calories or less. Now, that will do you wonders in case you're trying to lose weight.

Paleo Meatballs

This Paleo meatball recipe is easily filling. I usually just eat 3 or 4 of these and then I'm stuffed. You can make these meatballs under 10 minutes; great for quick lunches.

Ingredients:

- Meat (1 pound lean ground beef)
- Garlic (3 cloves)
- Parsley
- Onion (1 whole)
- Egg (1 regular egg)
- Almond meal (1 cup)
- *Your choice of spices*

Instructions:

Preheat oven to 400 degrees Fahrenheit. Mix garlic, parsley, and onion in food processor. Place all ingredients include the garlic mix in a bowl and then mix well until you achieve your preferred consistency. Form into meatballs – one meat ball should fit your hand. Bake meatballs for 20 minutes. Serve with a salad or any side dish.

Slow Cooked Ribs

Do you love pork ribs? I do. Here's a recipe for cooking pork ribs using a slow cooker. It's not every day when you can cook meat to perfection. Oh by the way, you can always substitute beef ribs if you're not too keen on pork.

Ingredients:

- Freshly milled black pepper
- Pork ribs (2 lbs.)

- White wine vinegar (¼ cup)
- Diced tomatoes (2 cans, BPA-free, no-salt added)
- Allspice (1 tablespoon)
- Carrots (4 pieces, cut into chunks)
- Turnips (4 pieces, cut into chunks)
- White onion (1 piece, large, sliced)
- ***Pressed garlic (4 cloves)***

Instructions:

Chop the rack of ribs into equal serving sizes (I use 2 ribs per piece). Cook ribs in medium heat for 10 minutes or until all sides have browned. Mix onions, garlic, allspice, vinegar, and tomatoes in slow cooker. Add browned ribs when everything has been well incorporated. Cook on low for 6 hours. Add turnips as well as the carrots after the first 5 hours of slow cooking. The meat should be quite tender when it's well-done (after 6 hours of slow cooking, that is).

Banana Bread On The Go

You can pre-cook this banana bread and keep it in the fridge so you have something that you can take with you in case you're always on the go. It's also a good solution for a quick lunch idea. The bread is exceptionally filling and the good news is that you can take as much as you want.

Ingredients:

- Eggs (3 pieces, regular size)
- Salt (just a pinch)
- Medium size ripe bananas (2 pieces, peeled and mashed)
- Raw honey (1 tbsp.)
- Vanilla Extract (1 tsp.)
- Coconut oil (2½ tbsps.)
- Desiccated coconut (2 tbsps.)
- Almond meal (1½ cup)
- Tapioca flour (2 tbsps)
- Cinnamon powder (1 tsp.)

- Nutmeg (just a pinch)
- Gluten free baking powder (1 tsp.)
- Walnuts (3 tbsp., chopped)
- ***Dried apricots (6 pieces, chopped)***

Instructions:

Preheat your oven to 340 degrees Fahrenheit. Line the bottom of a loaf tin with baking paper. Remember to brush it with coconut oil first. Break eggs into a mixing bowl. Season it with salt. Whisk them until foamy.

Mix in bananas, coconut oil, vanilla, and honey. Add coconuts, cinnamon, nutmeg, tapioca, baking powder, and almond meal. Fold in any dried fruit you want to add along with the walnuts. Smooth the surface.

Bake for 50 minutes. Remove from the oven when it's done and allow it to cool for 15 minutes. Slice into serving sizes. You can even pre-pack them, one for each day.

Sample Paleo Dinner Recipes

Dinners should cap your day and you should end it with a delectable meal. Some people like to eat heavy dinners while others just like something light. It all depends on your own personal preference and dietary needs.

Hunter Gatherer Stew

I often imagine myself as a modern-day hunter gatherer when I prepare this recipe. It's also a good way to cook any extra meat, veggies, and what not that's left at the end of the week. You're going to do your groceries tomorrow anyway so toss the rest of the things in the fridge into this stew (just kidding!).

Ingredients:

- Beef (cubed, 2 pounds)
- Red wine
- Onion (large, sliced)

- Salt
- Garlic powder
- Oregano
- Pepper
- Coconut oil
- Butter
- Carrots (small, sliced into lengths)
- ***Blueberries (a handful)***

Instructions:

Fry the beef in coconut oil until all sides are brown. Add onions and bring heat down to a simmer. Add all the seasoning. Add carrots. Add red wine for added flavor. Add water until everything is almost covered. Let it all simmer in medium heat for 20 minutes.

Add berries and butter. Simmer for another 10 minutes. Serve.

Paleo Pork Roast

I don't claim to be a gourmet chef but I think this is as gourmet as I have tried it to be. Apparently I don't have superb cooking skills. However, this recipe does prove that you don't have to be a gourmet cook to make really delectable meals. If I can do it, then anybody can.

Ingredients:

- Pork loin roast (3lbs., get the boneless ones)
- Garlic (5 cloves, minced)
- Ground cumin (2 tsp.)
- Black pepper (freshly ground)
- Paleo cooking fat (2 tbsp.)
- Chili powder (1 tbsp.)
- Sea salt
- Homemade stock (1 ½ cups)
- Onion (1 regular sized, thinly sliced)
- Bay leaves (2 pieces)

- Whole tomatoes (14oz can, get the one with juices)
- Ground coriander (2 tsp.)
- ***Apple cider vinegar (¼ cup)***

Instructions:

Season the pork roast with salt and pepper. Sear pork over medium heat. Use cooking fat on skillet when you sear the meat. Add cumin, coriander, onion, and garlic into the same skillet.

Add vinegar and allow it to boil. Wait until almost all of the liquid has evaporated. Add stock. Pour everything into a slow cooker, make sure to get all the drippings (this is the big secret!).

Add tomatoes along with the juices. Add bay leaves and adjust the seasoning to your liking. Set slow cooker to cook for 8 hours. You may remove the bay leaves before serving the dish.

Sample Paleo Snacks

The other good thing about going Paleo is that there are a lot of things to snack on. Sure you have to give up a lot of processed food, but you're getting something natural in exchange which also taste just as good.

Paleo Chocolate Bits

Now who says you have to give up on chocolate just to go Paleo on your diet? The only difference between the processed chocolate you can get from the store with the one in this recipe is the natural ingredients.

Ingredients:

- Cocoa powder (¾ cup)
- Coconut oil (¾ cup)
- Maple syrup (⅓ cup)
- Salt (⅛ teaspoon)
- ***Vanilla extract (1 teaspoon)***

Instructions:

Melt coconut oil using medium heat. Stir salt, honey, vanilla extract, and cocoa powder. Mix until the mixture obtains a smooth texture.

Pour chocolate mixture into a lined baking pan. Refrigerate for an hour. Chop into small bits (I like to cut them into bars – kids love it!). Store in fridge – serve as needed.

Banana Chips

This recipe is a personal favorite. These banana chips are really easy to make and they taste pretty good too.

Ingredients:

- Bananas (4 pieces, medium size)
- *Lemon juice*

Instructions:

Preheat oven to 200 degrees Fahrenheit. Slice the bananas – make slices as thin as possible. Coat the banana slices lightly in vinegar. Line a cookie sheet. Place banana slices on cookie sheet bake each side for 10 minutes or until each side is crispy.

Roasted Sweet Potatoes

If you're looking for a tastier alternative to the usual store bought fries then this recipe will not disappoint. The only downside I can see about this recipe is that it takes a bit of effort to chop the sweet potatoes into French fry wedges. Other than that, everything's pretty good!

Ingredients:

- Fresh ground cinnamon (1 tablespoon)
- Sweet potatoes (2 pieces, large)
- Virgin olive oil (2 tablespoons)
- *Salt*

Instructions:

Preheat oven to 350 degrees Fahrenheit. Peel and slice sweet potatoes into French fry wedges. Place in baking pan. Drizzle it with olive oil. Season to taste and add cinnamon if you wish.

Give it a light toss before baking. Bake for half an hour. Take the wedges out and turn them then bake the other side. Serve when both sides have a golden color.

Chapter 5: 3-Day Paleo Meal Plan

It is essential that you plan your meals ahead if you are starting on the Paleo diet. Beginners usually ask whether a certain recipe can be considered Paleo or not. Of course there are those who easily get comfortable with this diet – some can even come up with new recipes or just substitute Paleo ingredients for the non-Paleo ones.

But take things slowly. You can begin with the recipes mentioned earlier. As you look for more Paleo recipes you will soon get the hang of it.

Since not all beginners are expected to master the diet in so little a time, we have prepared a sample 3-day meal plan that you can follow. While following this basic meal plan you can look up some more Paleo recipes that you can add to this meal plan to make it last beyond the initial three days.

Reminders

- This meal plan assumes that you usually eat 3 regular meals each day. It is also assumed in the plan that you take at least one snack each day. However, do take note that you can adjust the time when you take the snack. If you don't like taking a snack then skip it or reserve that for another time.
- Serving sizes are all up to you. You should also check out the recipes for serving sizes as well if you're looking for new recipes; you can always add or reduce servings if you want to. If you feel that you want to have another helping then get another one.
- *If you want to substitute recipes make sure that you substitute lunch recipes with lunch recipes as well (dinner for dinner recipes and breakfast recipes for breakfast recipes).*

3-Day Paleo Meal Plan

Day 1:

- Breakfast: Stuffed Peppers
- Lunch: Paleo Meatballs
- Snack: Paleo Chocolate Bits
- ***Dinner: Hunter Gatherer Stew***

Day 2:

- Breakfast: English Muffins
- Lunch: Slow Cooked Ribs
- Snack: Banana Chips
- ***Dinner: Paleo Pork Roast***

Day 3:

- Breakfast: Eggs Benedict (or Paleo Pancakes if you fancy those)
- Lunch: Banana Bread on the Go
- Snack: Roasted Sweet Potatoes
- ***Dinner: (Pick your own preferred dinner)***

As you might have guessed, the recipes included in this meal plan come from the recipes mentioned in the previous chapter. You should also note that on day 3 of this meal plan, I have not specified any particular recipe.

I was hoping that by then you can make up your own mind and choose a dinner recipe of your own liking. Now, there are literally hundreds of Paleo recipes out there so don't just stick to the ones I have included here.

You can use the ones in this book to give you a place to start but you should take the initiative to find more recipes. The good news about this diet is that the modern Paleo community is a generous one. A lot of the folks who are into Paleo share their recipes and so you can say that you have a bountiful resource.